Eugene Eisenberg

Real-time in the brain limbic system

Eugene Eisenberg

Real-time in the brain limbic system
Translated from Russian by Inna Shragina-Mytnik

LAP LAMBERT Academic Publishing

Impressum / Imprint

Bibliografische Information der Deutschen Nationalbibliothek: Die Deutsche Nationalbibliothek verzeichnet diese Publikation in der Deutschen Nationalbibliografie; detaillierte bibliografische Daten sind im Internet über http://dnb.d-nb.de abrufbar.

Alle in diesem Buch genannten Marken und Produktnamen unterliegen warenzeichen-, marken- oder patentrechtlichem Schutz bzw. sind Warenzeichen oder eingetragene Warenzeichen der jeweiligen Inhaber. Die Wiedergabe von Marken, Produktnamen, Gebrauchsnamen, Handelsnamen, Warenbezeichnungen u.s.w. in diesem Werk berechtigt auch ohne besondere Kennzeichnung nicht zu der Annahme, dass solche Namen im Sinne der Warenzeichen- und Markenschutzgesetzgebung als frei zu betrachten wären und daher von jedermann benutzt werden dürften.

Bibliographic information published by the Deutsche Nationalbibliothek: The Deutsche Nationalbibliothek lists this publication in the Deutsche Nationalbibliografie; detailed bibliographic data are available in the Internet at http://dnb.d-nb.de.

Any brand names and product names mentioned in this book are subject to trademark, brand or patent protection and are trademarks or registered trademarks of their respective holders. The use of brand names, product names, common names, trade names, product descriptions etc. even without a particular marking in this work is in no way to be construed to mean that such names may be regarded as unrestricted in respect of trademark and brand protection legislation and could thus be used by anyone.

Coverbild / Cover image: www.ingimage.com

Verlag / Publisher:
LAP LAMBERT Academic Publishing
ist ein Imprint der / is a trademark of
OmniScriptum GmbH & Co. KG
Heinrich-Böcking-Str. 6-8, 66121 Saarbrücken, Deutschland / Germany
Email: info@lap-publishing.com

Herstellung: siehe letzte Seite /
Printed at: see last page
ISBN: 978-3-659-59235-5

Copyright © 2015 OmniScriptum GmbH & Co. KG
Alle Rechte vorbehalten. / All rights reserved. Saarbrücken 2015

Eugene Eisenberg

Real-time in Brain Limbic System

Content

Annotation	2
Introduction	3
The review of publications devoted to the brain limbic system	3
The Elements of the BLS information model	5
The BLS in the light of the Automatic Regulation and Control Theory	10
Impact via acupuncture points as a method for correcting the BLS	14
Neuron model	16
Delta modulator of the model	19
The work of the neuron model and physiological experiments	22
The perceptron with two-level memory and time slots of data processing	24
Sync generator of the neural network and its live prototype	34
Synchronization in neural networks	36
The period of cyclic activity of perception in time slots	38
Identification of time slots	40
Numerical evaluation of time slot activity (under weak perturbations)	43
Ability to handle EEG	45
The placement of the EEG electrodes	47
Analysis of impulse activity of the acupuncture points	48
Perceptron and physiological experiments	49
The General Conclusions	52
The Afterword	53
Reference	54
Real-time in Brain Limbic System (short description)	56

Annotation

The results of the suggested research were obtained in the course of the analysis of the descriptions of the brain limbic system's (BLS) morphological and functional structures. The author conducted a partial qualitative analysis of the BLS functions in order to create an analytical description, at least, of some of the BLS traits.

The inferred analytical expressions describe the behavior of any parameter of homeostasis. This provides the insight into various processes in the body.

Measuring these parameters at different time points with the following calculating of the coefficients of analytical expressions would allow to estimate the dynamics, to define the change obtained in the last time point (without performing any new measurements), and to make the forecast for the next time interval.

The performed analysis gave enough material to synthesize the model of teaching and memory in the BLS. This is a self-tuning phase-impulse system of regulation and operation.

The model of a neuron was synthesized as the basic building material for the BLS and it fits all the functions the BLS performs.

The analogy between the correction of transfer function of the phase-impulse system of regulation and operation (it is fulfilled by corrective chains) and the change in homeostasis (when acupuncture points are stimulated) has been found.

The model of a neuron was created with the following features: the ability to get adapted to various changes of input signals; the ability to get synchronized; the ability for spatial-time accumulating of a set of excitations; the possession of the mechanism of excitation and inhibition; the ability to process input information in time slots according to the phase of a corresponding receptor modality.

Optimal values were calculated for some electrical characteristics of the neuron model.

The comparison of the results received in the known electrophysiological experiments with the results obtained in the computer experiments, confirmed the adequacy of the model as the live system's prototype.

The author proposes the concept of a cyclic processing of neuron's receptor information in time slots every one of which corresponds to a particular receptor modality and to a certain phase of synchronization.

The synchronization parameters, which make this cycle possible, have been computed.

The information about the sources of synchronization in the living prototypes of such systems has been collected by reviewing the published works.

The synthesized model realizes the idea of time-sharing in the processing of information in the BLS.

The interval between regular time slots activities was defined and its approximate duration was analytically computed. The obtained results are sustained by the experimental data collected by physiologists.

Some ideas how to define a time slot's phase intended for processing information of different modalities have been proposed. To justify the existence of these time slots, the following conceptions were used: the holographic nature of the neural network and the informational exchange between living cells realized by coherent bio photons.

A method for carrying out the analysis of impulse activity of acupuncture points has been proposed.

Introduction

The work presented above in theses was carried out by the author in compliance with the contract signed with the organization Post Box P-6429 on 05.05.1983.

The research was approved by Resolution No.97 "On improving the diagnosis and treatment of lung diseases using new methods of information processing" from 04.07.1983 and it was jointly adopted by The Academy of Sciences of the USSR, The Academy of Medical Sciences, The Ministry of Health, and The Ministry of Electronic Industry.

The final report on the research was published just in 4 copies (1983) within the unadvertised company (Post Box P-6429) working for the Military Industry; therefore, this book has never really seen the light. With the edition at hand, the author tries to bridge the gap of the past. He also believes that the value of the results obtained then in the course of the work has not decreased and even, on the contrary, they might contribute a lot to the research works conducted in the field nowadays.

The review of publications devoted to the brain limbic system

The study of the brain limbic system (BLS) traditionally focuses on the structure of the brain, which is of a key importance for such issues as the implementation of motivational and emotional reactions and realization of learning and memory processes.

The scientific views on the structural and functional organization of the BLS have been formed under the influence of the classic works of Brown and Schaefer (1888), Holtz (1892), Woodworth and Sherrington (1904), Cannon and Britton (1925), Dyusser de Baren (1926) and Bard (1928). However, the work by Kluwer and Bucy (1939) is, definitely, the corner stone in the experimental studies while the work by Papez (1937) - in the theoretical studies in the field. Kluwer and Bucy studied the effect of damage of the temporal region of the neocortex and paleocortex on monkeys' behavior and reported about tremendous changes which manifested themselves in the fact that the monkeys became tame; namely, hypoactive and they also revealed such features as emotional dullness, blindness, loss of fear, aggression, and hyper sexuality.

The expert in brain anatomy, Papez (1937) questioned the traditional concept of highly specialized functions of the olfactory brain and put forward a new approach supposing that a large part of this system is included in the regulation of affective behavior but not the sense of smell.

On the base of the studies conducted by Brock (1878), Papez described a "circle" of interconnected neural structures consisting of gyrus cinguli, hippocampus, mammillary bodies and front thalamic nucleus, all of which are responsible for the appearance and flow of emotions.

Later, McLean (1949) broadened the borders of the Papez' theory by showing the important role of the BLS not only in the emotional behavior regulation but also in receiving and correcting internal and external signals entering the brain.

Subtle neurophysiological methods provide the results supporting the fact that, on one hand, there are important connections between the individual structures of the BLS and, on the other hand, there is a not-less-important connection between the BLS and the other systems of the brain, such as the reticular formation, basal ganglia, and neocortex (Vinogradova, 1975, Science, 1960).

Many different methods were used to study the functional organization of the BLS and its individual units. Here are some of those methods:
- To study the effect of limbic structure damage on the behavior;
- To study the effect of the direct electrical and chemical stimulation of limbic structures;
- To study the dynamics of BLS electrical activity patterns detected during different behavioral acts;

The method of studying the effects of BLS structures damage revealed the involvement of these BLS structures into the creation of motivational and emotional behavior as well as into the regulation of learning and memorizing processes [24, p.42].

The analysis of autonomic, somatic, and behavioral effects caused by electrical and chemical stimulating of various BLS structures in many respects, supplements the data collected via the method based on the BLS structures damage.

The contradictory facts, which often might be found in the publications, can be explained in most cases by a definite shortcoming of the method of direct stimulation (especially, electrical stimulation) of brain structures.

An extremely small size of the anatomically separate cores of such structures as hypothalamus, amygdala, septum, thalamus, etc. interferes with their selective activation – the annoying current spreads over the neighboring areas. As a result, it is very difficult to correlate the effect produced by the excitation of a specific nerve structure with the structure itself.

The method of chemical stimulation was proved to give more reliable results: first, certain doses of physiologically active substances (the mediators of synaptic transmission) may not be involved into excitation pathways; second, such doses can selectively excite those nerve populations that have only relevant synaptic chemo-sensitivity [24].

The analysis of the neurons' impulse activity, which takes place in different formations and in the BLS peripherals in response to external signals of different modalities, in particular, to the light signals, is found to be especially valuable.

The most important feature of the BLS is, that it integrates the ability to receive information about both the external environment and shifts of the internal environment. This enables the BLS to inform the brain integrating systems of arising biological needs.

After the information has been identified and processed, the BLS can run autonomic, somatic, and behavioral responses via its efferent connections. These processes provide both the adaptation of the organism to the environment and preservation of the optimal level of the internal environment. This is exactly one of the main functions of the BLS.

The most complete list of the publications devoted to the issues related to the BLS is presented in [24], p.441.

Though the morphology of the BLS will need to be further studied, quite a clear picture of bilateral nerve connections between its various levels and structures has been built already.

In the following chapters, the existing information about the BLS will be used as the basis for constructing a hypothetical model of the BLS functionality.

The Elements of the BLS information model

The description of the limbic system of cats' brain created by Vinogradova is, probably, the most convenient one to start the analysis with (see Vinogradova [1], p.256). In the experiment run by Vinogradova, the finest electrodes were implanted into each of the known core limbic system. Flashes were produced at irregular intervals affecting the visual system of the cats. All the impulses, which were produced simultaneously with the core signals' input and output, were thoroughly recorded.

Figure 1 shows the limbic system which served as the basis for the analysis. In order to reach a full picture of the phenomenon, more factors affecting the BLS system are to be introduced into the analysis. As a result, the following components were added to the system:
- the peripherals comprising the variety of all body tissues including external receptors (they realize the constant watch over the changes in the outside world) and internal receptors (they perform tracing after the internal changes of the organism);
- efferent and afferent pathways of spinal cord;
- endocrine glands;

- the circulatory system;
- the lymphatic system.

To perform the analysis in a more efficient way, each block of the scheme presented in Figure 1 is built of different pieces of functionality, which are morphologically connected with each other. The analysis of the scheme contributes to understanding of the properties of the BLS system as a system of regulation.

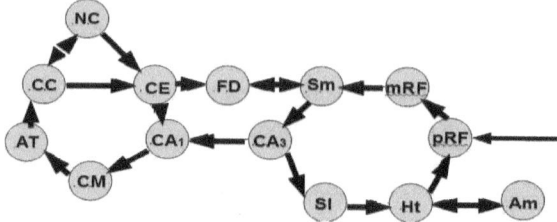

Figure 1: Scheme of the basic interactions between the structural elements of the limbic system.

The cores in the circles of Papez:
CA_1, CA_3 – fields of hippocampus; FD – gyrus dentatus; Sm, Sl – medial and lateral septum nucleus; mRf, pRf – mesencephalic and pontobulbar nucleus of the reticular formation; Ht – hypothalamus;
Am – amygdala; CM – mammillary bodies; AT – front (limbic) thalamic nucleus; CC, CE – cingulate gyrus and entorhinal limbic cortex; NC – neocortex.

According to a vast group of neurophysiologists, CA_3, a field of hippocampus, compares the information of the gyrus dentatus (FD) with the medial septum nucleus (Sm). This comparison takes places at fixed time intervals [1] and it synchronizes the connections, especially, between the septum and gyrus dentatus. The phenomenon of synchronization in a neural network is the fact recognized by some other studies. For example, it is stated in 'Bionics'[2] that "the mechanisms of external synchronization of neurons is synchronized under the influence of individual pacemakers" ([2], p.103). This and many other studies prove the existence of external synchronization of neurons; however, the interaction between the pacemakers is not clear yet.

According to [1], p.257, the field of hippocampus, CA_3, transmits signals of visual information only of a certain narrow range of frequencies. However, the same result will be achieved (the authors of the work did not pay attention to this fact), if the visual information is processed by the BLS in certain repeated phase intervals (time slots). Every phase is connected to a fixed point within the synchronization period.

Hence, the following statements are essential:
- synchronization exists;
- the responses are regularly generated to the visual stimulation signals whose frequency is limited by the range of 10-30 Hz.

In the text, the term "time slot" stands for a time interval when the information, which has been received from neuro receptors of a particular modality, is processed. This interval is associated with a certain phase of the sync frequency. The time slot will be called active if the corresponding information is being processed during this interval.

Since visual and any other sensory information is processed by the same BLS blocks, it is appropriate to assume, that processing of signals of different modality (by the same structural units) requires the processes to be shifted in time.

The output mismatch signal CA_3 allows the information to pass through from the entorhinal part of the limbic cortex CE to the mammillary bodies CM via the hippocampus field CA_1.

It is necessary to pay attention to the fact that hippocampus CA_1, mammillary bodies CM, frontal (limbic) nucleus of the thalamus and cingulate gyrus CC, which are sequentially connected in the left circle of Papez' scheme, do not let the input signals through, after the signals' first occurrence – more occurrences are required.

For the convenience of use, let us call the spatial-timing sequence of impulses by Image. Then, the characteristic of each block mentioned above can be described with the simple engineering language as follows:
- Online Image (oI) is stored in the buffer memory (similar to clipboard function);
- The number of oI occurrences is accumulated in the counter of the block (the number of input signal occurrences, which are necessary for an appropriate output signal to be released, varies among the mentioned blocks from 2 to 10 times);
- After the output signal (oI) has been released from the clipboard, the buffer counter returns to its original state (similar to a reset operation);
- In the BLS blocks CA_1, CM, AT, and CC, after the shape of the input has been changed, the form of the response to the original input signal remains the same for some period, which is defined by the number of input signal occurrences required in a particular block, for perceiving the change.

Figure 2 shows a more detailed version of the synthesized scheme presented above in Figure 1. It is an obvious fact that, the extent to which the BLS scheme might be broken down into details, totally depends on the level of knowledge about the functions of its structures and their morphological inter relations. Starting the discussion of the regulatory system scheme (which is the version of the BLS scheme presented in Figure 1), it is important to note that the hippocampal field CA_1 bears the form of a logical ban scheme. Unlike this, in computing technique with only two states (open and closed), the scheme at hand partially transmits the signal to the mammillary bodies CM in the case when no complete coincidence of the compared signals is detected.

The transmitted signal corresponds to the newness of the input oI compared to the information which has been released from the long term memory NC and sent to the input of comparator assigned to one of the hippocampus CA_3 fields.

It is worth mentioning the probabilistic character of the necessary number of input signal (oI) occurrences, required for the blocks of two Papez' circles, in order to activate a corresponding output.

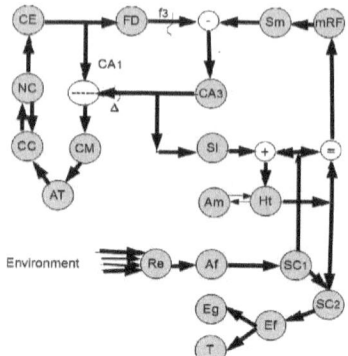

Figure 2: Limbic system after logical transformations

The added blocks: Ef, Af - efferent and afferent nervous systems; T, Re - the collection of tissues and receptors; SC_1, SC_2 - afferent and efferent pathways of spinal cord; Eg - endocrine glands (they sustain the biochemical communication with all the parts of the brain's limbic system via the bloodstream).

The blocks forming the circle of Papez, work with the outputs of hippocampal field CA_1 in a synchronous way. In other words, processing of visual information is performed in strict time slots with their particular starting points (phases) in relation to the period of synchronization in the BLS.

The phase of the signal emerging (in hippocampal field CA_1) in the response to coming visual information, does not depend on the duration and duty cycle of light flashes.

Since each of the BLS blocks performs the spatial-timing conversion of an input signal, it would be reasonable to divide them further into sub-blocks, the converters.

The phenomenon of input signal transformation might be characterized via bringing up a quote from Gelfand and Tsetlin [3]: "...the purpose of each conversion – reduction of the redundancy of the transmitted information" (p.57). This is, apparently, relevant for biological systems at all levels.

Due to the existing information delay, a signal released from the CA_1 hippocampus field reaches the neocortex NC only after some repeated signal occurrences have taken place at CA_1. Then, the "new picture" is identified in the neocortex that is similar to the act of transferring data from RAM to the long-term memory.

"The sequential signals that are similar in configuration may cause (in the neocortex) residual cumulative effects, either by putting in order accidental chains of macromolecules, or by increasing their excitability; therefore, this area responds more easily to the repetition of the same stimulation" (Pribram [4]). Analyzing the BLS scheme, it is important to note that gyrus dentatus FD plays the role of buffer memory, whose function is to register the modified Image contained in the neocortex for the purposes of further comparing it by the hippocampus CA_3. The reflection of the newest part of the image, circulates in the left circle of Papez' scheme. This reflection is updated with the information from the hippocampus.

The Papez' circles resemble RAM on delay ring lines in computer facilities. Not unlike the unchangeable binary impulse sequences circulating in delay ring lines of computer engineering, the spatial timing image, which circulates in the circles of Papez, is more complex than any binary sequence and it is continuously modified.

One more time, the found parallel confirms the view of Koehler [3], that there is a well-known isomorphism between the brain and other physical devices.

Considering the other Papez' circle, it is important to emphasize that a signal released by the hippocampus CA_3, is split and a part of it is directed to the septum SI lateral nucleus which plays the role of inertial unit, according to the findings of electrophysiological experiments [1]. From the septum SI lateral nucleus, the signals go further to the hypothalamus Ht, which also percepts the signals from the spinal cord afferents SC_1. The signals from the spinal cord afferents SC_1 bear the information about the external world, which is collected by periphery exterior receptors, as well as the information about the status of the body collected by inter receptors (temperature, osmotic pressure of blood, carbon dioxide level in blood, glucose level, etc.).

A set of receptors (Re) are controlled by signals emitted by the hypothalamus (Ht) and sent through afferent pathways of the spinal cord (SC_2), efferent nervous system (pRf), and tissue (T). Pontobulbar (pRf) and mesencefalic (mRf) nuclei of the reticular formation, reveal the newness of a stimulus and submit the information on this newness to the septum medial nucleus (Sm).

The nuclei of the hypothalamus (Ht) affect the endocrine glands (Eg) which, in their turn, produce biologically active substances (hormones and some others) which are spread with the blood and lymph throughout the body including all the nuclei of the limbic system. This chemical link is not shown in Figure 2 to avoid overloading of the scheme.

The details of physical realization of the "elementary" blocks (see Figure 2), some functions of which are found to be parallel with some known technical devices, remain mostly obscure. However, the electrophysiological descriptions [1] allow assuming that there are some parts of the BLS which fulfill the functions presented by the technical symbols in Figure 2.

The model of a neuron is the basic element of the BLS, which allows the realization of all the functions presented in Figure 2. This is discussed below in the dedicated chapter.

The model of perceptron is based on the mentioned basic neuronal elements and it preserves the working characteristics of the BLS. The model is discussed in chapter "The perceptron with two-level memory and time slots of data processing".

Conclusion

Referring to the existing publications on the morphological and functional structures of the BLS, the author has performed a partial analysis of the BLS operating.

The BLS in the light of the Automatic Regulation and Control Theory

Let us consider the diagram in Figure 2 from some specific positions.
The homeostasis of the organism is operated by the regulating impulse (binary) sequences, which influence the work of heart, blood system, control centers, etc. These impulses also affect various endocrine glands, triggering them to produce active biochemical catalysts.

Assuming tha,t all the BLS neurons treat information of one modality during its fixed phase interval (time slot), which is located within the period of synchronizing frequency, we will cut the impulses of this phase out of all impulse sequences in the BLS. The frequency of the cut out impulses f(t) will serve as the output parameter of the analyzed system.

Based on the previous statements, the scheme (Figure 2) may be upgraded by marking out a self-tuning circuit (STC) and an auto-regulation circuit (ARC) in it.
Then, STC includes blocks Sl, Ht, Am, pRF, and CA_3 while ARC includes blocks CA_1, CM, AT, CC, NC, CE, and FD (see Figure 1).

When the ARC part of the system, with its responses to weak short-term influences of the environment, is the subject of the study, the communication via connection CA_3- NC may be neglected due to the known fact that signals get from CA_3 to the input of NC only in the result of frequently repeated stimuli.
As reaction NC is an unknown function of the information arrived to this block from all the parts of the body, it is possible to specify the NC entrance's influence on comparator CA_3 with the arbitrary function of time $f_3(t)$.
Figure 2 has been adjusted for the purpose of studying the influence of weak short term impacts and its new version is presented in Figure 3. The connection between the signals can be expressed in operator forms:

$$W_{SC1}(W_{Af}(W_{rl}(u(t)))) - f(t) = \delta(t) \qquad (1)$$
$$f(t) = W_{Ht}(W_{Sl}(W_{Sm}(W_{mRf}(\delta(t))))) + W_{SC1}(W_{Af}(W_{Re}(u(t)))) \qquad (2)$$

where $f_3(t)$ – a signal from block FD. If this signal is missing, all the information from block Sm proceeds to block Sl.

f(t) - a signal from block Ht. This signal plays the role of a control vector of the regulation system.

u(t) - a signal simulating the impact of the environment on the system.

G(t) - a vector expressing the quantitative change of the hormone spectrum in the body with time (the number of vector's components complies with the types of hormones while the vector component's value depends on the amount of hormone of a certain type).

δ(t) - a signal from block pRf.

W_x - an operator of data transformation in block x. The designation of any block (Figure 3) may be substituted for "x".

The following assumption might be a good asset in performing the qualitative analysis:

For weak perturbations, the transfer function of any block in Figure 3 is created out of many linear functions such as amplifying, integrating, differentiating, inertial, oscillating, and summarizing. The nonlinear blocks in the input signals range, which is under study, can be considered as linear ones.

$$W_{SC1}(p)*W_{Af}(p)*W_{Re}(p)*u(p) - f(p) = \delta(p) \quad (3)$$

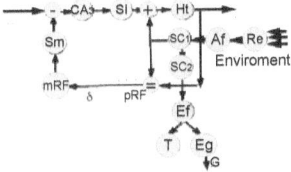

Figure 3: The BLS fragment of Figure 2 used for the analysis of weak perturbation

$$f(p)=W_{Ht}*(W_{Sl}(p)*W_{Sm}(p)*W_{mRf}(p)*\delta(p)+W_{SC1}(p)*W_{Af}(p)*W_{Re}(p)*u(p) \quad (4)$$

Denote:
$$W_{SAR}(p) = W_{SC1}(p)*W_{Af}(p)*W_{Re}(p) \quad (5)$$
$$W_{SSM}(p) = W_{Sl}(p)*W_{Sm}(p)*W_{mRf}(p) \quad (6)$$

Then, we get
$$W_{SAR}(p)*U(p) - f(p) = \delta(p) \quad (7)$$
$$F(p) = W_{Ht}(p)*(W_{SSM}(p)*\delta(p) + W_{SAR}(p)*U(p)) \quad (8)$$

where $W_x(p)$ is a Carson-Heaviside transform of transfer function W_x.

f(p), δ(p), u(p) – Carson-Heaviside transforms of f(t), δ(t), and u(t) respectively.

By solving the system (7, 8), we get the expression for transfer function of the system (with zero initial conditions).

$$\Phi(p) = f(p)/u(p) = W_{SAR}(p)*W_{Ht}(p)*(1 + W_{SSM}(p))/(1 + W_{Ht}(p) * W_{SSM}(p)) \quad (9)$$

The desired transfer function we are looking for presents the reaction of the system to a single stepwise signal.

Therefore, transition function of the system can be obtained as a result of the inverse Carson-Heaviside transform of transfer function of the closed system (9).

Note that Carson-Heaviside transform $\Phi(p)$ in (9) can be represented in general case as $\Phi(p) = B(p)/D(p) = \Sigma_i b_i * p^{m-i} / \Sigma_j a_j * p^{n-j}$ (10)

where i=0,..m; j=0,..,n;

whereas m < n and equation D(p) does not have zero roots.

Then, the general solution to the differential equation, which describes the behavior of the ARC system, has form (11).

$\Phi_o(t) = \Sigma_i (\Sigma_j (C_{ij} * t^j) * e^{\lambda_i t})$ (11)

where i=1,..m; j=0,..,k_j-1;

$\lambda_1, \lambda_2,.., \lambda_m$ - different roots of the characteristic equation $D(\lambda) = 0$;

$k_1, k_2,..k_m$ - their multiplicity where $\Sigma_i k_i = N$.

With this, a weak dependence of coefficients C_{ij}, λ_i on time is allowed that is a characteristic of a healthy individual. The system is stable if there are no positive real parts among λ_i. The time graphs of the desired transition function described by (11) are presented in Figure 4 (b, c, and d).

4a corresponds to the disturbance at the input of ARC;

4b, 4c, 4d present the ARC system reactions to a weak short-term disturbance for different values λ_i.

It is important to note that any specification of morphological or other links in the ARC scheme (Figure 3) in combination with preserving of feedback does not change the nature of the general solution of differential equations describing the behavior of the ARC.

Note that the theoretical graphics b, c, and d (Figure 4) reflect the known experimental data in a qualitative way, for example, the dynamics of blood pressure p(t) for a healthy person when suddenly his/her physical activity L(t) is increased and maintained for some time.

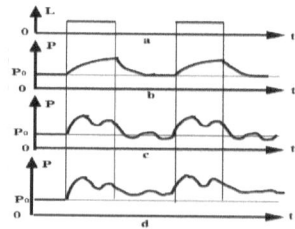

Figure 4: Possible responses of blood pressure to any disturbing factor

The other parameters of homeostasis, which characterize the live regulation system, would produce graphs of the same character in response to the disturbing factors applied to them.

Generally speaking, equation (11) serves for describing even "badly" working systems of regulation.

Depending on the c_{ij} and λ_i values, short-term disturbances may lead to one of the following outcomes in the system: the transition process with a big-value time constant; or long time fluctuations; or overloading of the regulation system, i.e. the combination of c_{ij} and λ_i change and an "overloading" disturbance may result in a damage to the system.

Considering the issue of blood pressure fluctuation, it should be mentioned that, in a prolonged stressful situation which causes the blood pressure to increase, the need in increased blood pressure is memorized (see the information chain in the left Papez' circle, Figure 2).

Persistent attempts of the system to comply with the new arterial pressure level within both the servo system formed by the left Papez' circle and the comparing scheme CA_3, lead to the continuous transitional process around the shifted "normal" pressure. This mechanism manifests itself in the phenomenon of blood pressure instability in hypo- and hypertensive patients.

The sustainability of any regulation and control system, including the one under study may be analyzed on the base of the known block parameters by the methods designed for automatic control systems.

In theory, it is possible to determine the limits of parameter changes (for each block), which would not cause any disruption of the sustainability of the system as a whole.

Note that, the violation of the sustainability of the system is equal to the failure of the system. The knowledge of the numeric values of the regulation system parameters would enable to fix the system in the way that it will stay out of the range of instability.

The following are the main findings of the chapter:

1. There is synchronization in the work of all blocks in the limbic system.
2. The processing of visual information occurs in certain phases in relation to a given frequency.
3. In the working range of regulation, the change of parameters of homeostasis in time (only for weak perturbations) happens according to the law $\Sigma_i \Sigma_j (C_{ij} * t^j) * e^{\lambda_i t}$

   where $i=1,..m$; $j=0,...,k_j-1$;
   $\lambda_1, \lambda_2,..., \lambda_m$ - various roots of characteristic equation $D(\lambda) = 0$
   $k_1, k_2,..k_m$ - their multiplicity rates where $\Sigma_i k_i = N$
   N – order of the system.

Conclusion

The morphological and functional structures of the BLS were recreated as extremely truncated due to the limited knowledge in the field. The creation of the BLS structure pursued the purpose to describe analytically, at least, some of its properties.

The resulting analytical expressions, which describe behavior in the time of any parameter of homeostasis, provide the instrument for judging the dynamics of various processes in an organism.

Getting the values of these parameters at various time points, it is possible to make the assessment of the dynamics through calculating the coefficients of an analytical expression. For example, Figure 4 shows a possible character of parameters change affected by load L(t): aperiodic process (b), slowly fading oscillatory (c), not fading oscillatory process (d).

The change of the process dynamics may occur in the result of some event taken place in time point t_0 (taking a medicine or stopping a treatment, other types of therapy, some load).

Having calculated the coefficients of the obtained analytical expressions, it is possible to implement inter- and extrapolation, i.e. to evaluate the changes produced during the passed interval without performing measurements, and to forecast the future changes.

By connecting the changes in process dynamics, which take place at time t_0, with the complex of therapeutic procedures carried out at particular time, it is possible to estimate their meaning for an organism in a more precise way.

For example, frequent measuring of some blood parameters enables to see the difference in the recovery processes in postoperative patients proceeding at the background of taking or canceling this or that medicine.

According to the author, the new result of the chapter relates to the analytical presentation (see equation 11) of homeostasis parameters changes in time.

Impact via acupuncture points as a method for correcting the BLS

In impulse systems of automatic control and regulation, where coding of operating signals is performed by frequency or phase changing methods, the desired change of transfer function is achieved with the help of corrective chains.

The diagram of the elementary system of regulation with the feedback is presented in Figure 5 (a).
The diagram includes the following symbols:
W – transfer function of an open system,
W_{oc} – transfer function of the feedback block,
k – transfer coefficient of the system as a whole,
U_{in} – input signal,

U_{out} – output signal,
U_{oc} – feedback signal,
U_{cor} – corrective signal.

The validity of the following equations is evident for scheme (a):

$$U_{out} = (U_{in} - U_{oc}) * W \qquad (1)$$
$$U_{oc} = U_{out} * W_{oc} \qquad (2)$$
$$k = U_{out} / U_{in} = W / (1 + W * W_{oc}) \qquad (3)$$

Scheme (b) might be useful for performing the correction of scheme (a). The generator of corrective impulses sends the impulses to the block of comparison via the scheme of summation (integration) located in the feedback circuit. If corrective impulses are activated, the transfer function of the system changes its value.

By analogy with the above:

$$U_{out} = (U_{in} - (U_{cor} + U_{oc})) * W \qquad (4)$$
$$U_{oc} = U_{out} * W_{oc} \qquad (5)$$
$$k = U_{out} / U_{in} = W * (1 - U_{cor}) / (1 + W * W_{oc}) \qquad (6)$$

In case of simultaneous correction from multiple inputs, expression (6) may be transformed into

$$k = U_{out} / U_{in} = W * (1 - \Sigma_i a_i * U_{cor\,i}) / (1 + W * W_{oc}) \qquad (7)$$

where a_i - weight factors of each correcting input.

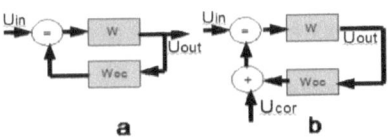

Figure 5: Block diagram of the control system (a - without correction, b - with correction)

In the BLS (as the system of regulation and control), neurons of reticular formation, which are connected to all receptors in an organism including the ones located in zones of acupuncture points, play the role of the integrator accepting the correcting signals.

The mentioned receptor neurons generate corrective impulses after they have been excited by an acupuncture needle or by any other way.

The repeating identical impacts on acupuncture points, cause the renewal of the transfer function value, which is stored at the beginning in RAM, realized in Papez' circles and, then, on the "hard disc" (this is parallel to recording in the neocortex) if the number of stimulus occurrences exceeds a threshold.

It should be taken into consideration, that the recurring impacts via acupuncture points may also lead to an undesirable change of transfer function value, for example, at a wrong diagnosis or at choosing wrong points of influence.

Since Paul Nogier introduced a new practice, doctors have been successfully treating different organs and systems by transmitting electric impulses with adjusted individual frequency to the corresponding acupuncture points of an auricle.

In fact, the effect is obtained owing to both the frequency influence and the phase impact (not only to the frequency influence): the impulses of different frequencies are superimposed on activity phases of different time slots. Knowing precisely the phase of synchronizing frequency, which conforms to the activity of a particular system in the body, we can influence this system in a more efficient way.

Conclusion.

This chapter shows the analogy between the correction of the transfer function of phase-impulse regulation system with the help of corrective chains and the change of homeostasis in the result of an impact applied to acupuncture points.

Neuron model

Despite the great morphological and functional diversity of real neurons, their formalized working processes reveal a number of common properties:

1) a neuron has multiple inputs and one output,
2) all inputs and the only output have just two states: "switch on" and "switch off",
3) a neuron becomes active when the algebraic sum of exciting and inhibiting signals exceeds a threshold,
4) in a neuron, signals move only in one direction.

Until now, the four properties listed above have characterized a so-called formal neuron or known also as a logical threshold element. If a network is built up with these neurons, its work will comply with the laws of Boolean algebra. However, Boolean algebra does not take into account the dynamics of the information treatment processes. From this point of view, a physiological (an informal one) neuron is an incomparably more complex structure. A live neuron shares the common properties (listed above) with a formal neuron and, in addition, it is characterized by the following traits:

5) the presence of absolute and relative refractory period,
6) the ability for adaptation,
7) the dependence of neuron's frequency of responses on the magnitude of an exciting signal
8) spatial-timing summation of multiple excitations is performed under neuron's synaptic mechanism control
9) the ability to create new sensory inputs and to destruct the part of the old inputs (the nature of the both phenomena has not been studied)

and some others.

Since the last three properties have not been comprised into any known formal model of neuron, the author tried to create a model which would embrace the both groups of properties, 1-4 and 6-8.

Since the BLS is a neural network (as it was mentioned earlier), a new model of neuron with the BLS properties named in the conclusion of the previous chapter looks as follows:

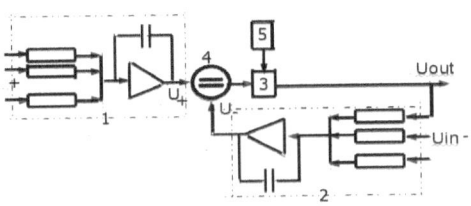

Figure 6: Neuron model

The scheme contains: 1 – the first memory block (integrator), 4 - block of comparison, 3 – block of coincidence, 2 – the second memory block (integrator of feedback), 5 – the generator of synchronizing impulses (external in relation to neurons).

A schematic representation of the excitation summing up in the synapse between the presynaptic fiber and the body of a ganglion cell, which served as the basis for the synthesis of the neuron model, is shown in Figure 7 ([9] p. 81).

The impulses coming to the inputs of integrators (see Figure 6, blocks 1 and 2) correspond to the impulses of presynaptic fiber presented in Figure 7.

The charge accumulated on the capacity of the feedback integrator (Figure 6, block 2) corresponds to the potential of a sub-synaptic membrane.

The output impulse sequence of the neuron model corresponds to the impulses of a postsynaptic fiber.

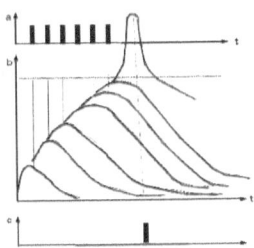

Figure 7: Summation of impulses at a neuron's input

a – the presynaptic fiber (potential for action)
b – the synapse (potential of a sub-synaptic membrane)
c – the postsynaptic fiber (potential for action)

Blocks of memory (1) and (2) are the most convenient to be realized on multiport integrators; though, in a live neuron, the place of the feedback integrator (2) is occupied by an element similar to a long RC-chain [9]. It is expected that replacing the RC-chain with an integrator in the working range of frequencies will not lead to significant distortions in the processing of the input data; to the opposite, this will noticeably facilitate the model realization in its arrangement, algorithm and the program.

The inputs of the both integrators serve as information inputs of neuron model. In the block of comparison, signals from integrators are marked with different algebraic symbols; therefore, one input will be considered as excitatory, while the other – inhibitory (maintaining the traditional neurophysiological terminology).

The output of the block of coincidence (3) serves as an information output of the model. This output lets the impulses of the generator (5) pass through if there is a permitting signal from the block of comparison (2).

The block of comparison (4) releases a permitting signal directed to block (3) only in the case if the inequality $U_- < U_+$ is true,

where U_+ - a signal from the integrator (1) output,

U_- - a signal from the output of the feedback integrator (2).

Hence, the impulse sequences arriving to the first block of memory (1) are summed up and form an analogue signal proceeding to the comparison circuit (4).

At the same time, the output impulse sequence and the input signals arriving at the input of the second block of memory (2), are summed up to form an analogue signal proceeding to the second input of the block of comparison (4).

If the value of a signal from the first block of memory (1) exceeds the value of the signal from the second memory block (2), the comparison block (4) produces a permitting signal and sends it to the coincidence circuit (3). The block of coincidence (3) may let or not let impulses from the generator of synchronizing impulses (5) pass through: this depends on the condition of the permitting input.

The generator of synchronizing impulses (5) is not a part of the neuron model, but it serves for synchronizing the neurons, which are included into the network of any structure. The mechanism of synchronization is discussed in the chapters "Sync generator of the neural network and its live prototype" and "Synchronization in neural networks".

Conclusion

The resulting model of a neuron, in addition to the properties of the predecessor models, has a number of new features:

- adaptation to the input signal changes, owing to the existence of corresponding feedback,
- ability for synchronizing,

- existence of the mechanisms of excitation and inhibition,
- the ability to process multi modality data: the data of every sensor modality is processed by turns in individual time micro intervals (time slots),
- the minimal number of elements.

Delta modulator of the model

It is important to note that analogue digital conversion in the model is similar to the corresponding conversion in delta modulator.

The following variables are to be introduced:

τ – the time constant of feedback integrator (τ will be defined below).

T – the period of synchronizing impulses (SI)

H - the amplitude of synchronizing impulses (we assume that the block of coincidence does not change the value of this amplitude when it lets an impulse pass through to the input of the feedback integrator).

Figure 8 shows the growth (of a saw tooth type) of signal $U_.(t)$ when there is a continuous series of impulses at the integrator's input (for simplicity, we assume that only one input of the feedback integrator is activated - the one which follows the block of coincidence (3) in Figure 6).

The right part of the same figure presents an exponential decrease in the values of $U_.(t)$ in the case when there are no impulses at the input of the integrator.

Obviously, the value of the function $U_.(t)$ increases, when τ increases, and the value decreases, when there are no signals at the input of the integrator.

On the other hand, the maximum rate of discharge of the capacity in the feedback integrator will take place when $\tau \rightarrow 0$. In this case the capacity does not preserve the charge and the charge accumulation becomes impossible.

In particular cases, delta modulator parameters for analog-digital conversions in a neuron could be defined in compliance with the character of occurring input signals (if the character is known). However, for the cases when the character of signals is unknown, the optimal value of τ should satisfy the condition of the equality of the average rate of capacity charging, when there is a continuous impulse sequence at one input, and the average discharge rate of the same capacity, when there are no impulses at the modulator's input.

Discharging of the capacity will take time equal to 3τ that is not enough to reduce the capacity's value up to zero.

Let A be the maximal value of signal $U_.(t)$.

We assume that the cutting front of the impulse at hand is so small that it can be neglected, i.e. steps of the saw instantly reach height H in the moment when the impulse arrives.

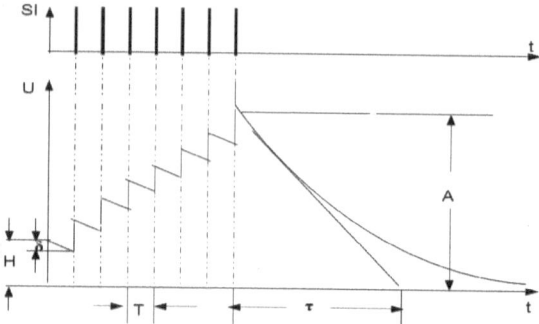

Figure 8: Time diagram of the delta modulator work in the neuron model

The function of capacity discharging varies in compliance with the $He^{-t/\tau}$ law. During the time equal to the period T of impulse arriving, the capacity gets discharged up to value $He^{-T/\tau}$. Hence, at a continuous set of charging impulses, during time T (one step in the graph), capacity's voltage will increase by the value

$$\Delta = H (1 - e^{-T/\tau}) \quad (1)$$

The average rate of voltage growing in a capacity is equal to

$$H (1 - e^{-T/\tau})/T \quad (2)$$

As a result, if max $dU_-(t)/dt$ is presented as V^+ and condition (3) is true

$$H (1 - e^{-T/\tau})/ T >= V^+ \quad (3)$$

then the neuron's delta-modulator is never late in tracing a changing input signal. Hence, the boundary value of τ is

$$\tau = T/\ln(V^+T - H) \quad (4)$$

The further increase of τ value at a given V^+ is meaningless.

Denote the maximal reduction rate of function $U_-(t)$ through V^- ($V^- <= 0$).

Then, for the best tracking of a decreasing signal on an input of neural delta-modulator, condition (5) will be true

$$V^- >= - A_0/ e^{-t/\tau} \quad (5)$$

where A_0 - the voltage of the capacity at the beginning of discharge.

After transformation, it looks

$$|V^-/A_0| <= e^{-t/\tau}/\tau \quad (6)$$

If the scope of functions is defined as $t \in [0, k\tau]$, the worst conditions to perform inequality (6) are provided in point $t = k\tau$.

Then, condition (7) is required to be fulfilled

$$\ln |V^-/A_0| \leq -k - \ln \tau \qquad (7)$$

To provide the tracking of a falling signal $U^-(t)$ on all interval $[0, k\tau]$ performed by delta-modulator, we transform (7) and get

$$e^{k+\ln|V^-/A_0|} \leq 1/\tau \qquad (8)$$

$$\tau \leq 1/e^k |V^-/A_0| = |A_0/V^-| e^{-k} \qquad (9)$$

Thus, we get the following bounds for the value of τ:

$$T/\ln(V^+T - H) \leq \tau \leq |A_0/V^-| e^{-k} \qquad (10)$$

where A_0 and k may be specified as parameters.

If inequality (10) is not fulfilled, the neuron's modulator delays in tracing a promptly changing input signal.

Let the rate of change of the input signal V^+ and V^- be unknown, then the optimal value τ will be determined taking into consideration the following:

MC - mathematical expectation for the input signal value.

Figure 9 shows the case when the input signal of the neuron's delta modulator is equal to the constant MC.

The best tracking of a constant signal on a modulator input will occur when the voltage on an integrator output (formed after the arrival of a new impulse) falls during time 2T to the voltage value which has been on this integrator output before the mentioned impulse arrives.

Since the integrator output voltage decreases exponentially $(MC + H/2) e^{-t/\tau}$, the following equality is true:

$$(MC + H/2) e^{-2T/\tau} = MC - H/2 \qquad (11)$$

This implies $\quad e^{-2T/\tau} = (MC - H/2)/(MC + H/2) \qquad (12)$

Taking the logarithm, we get

$$\tau = 2T/\ln((MC + H/2)/(MC - H/2)) \qquad (13)$$

Conclusion

As it is shown, the frequency of the output impulses in a steady state (when the selection of electrical characteristics is optimal in relation to the range of input signals variety) will be half the value of synchronization frequency.

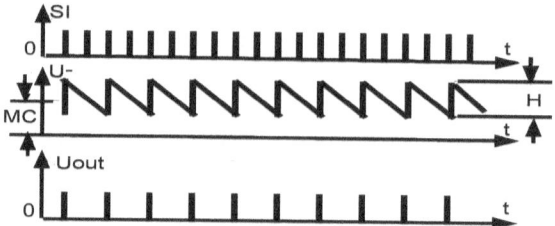

Figure 9: Delta modulator with constant input signals
SI – synchronizing impulses,
H – amplitude of an impulse,
MC – average value of a signal on the output of the feedback integrator,
U$_{out}$ – signal on an output delta-modulator.

The work of the neuron model and physiological experiments

It is interesting to compare the behavior of the synthesized model of neuron with the published descriptions of the behavior of the live prototype of the model which is a neural cell influenced by different kinds of inputs.

In electrophysiological experiments, the thinnest electrode was implanted into the body of an axon. The signals from the electrode were recorded together with the registration input signals. The experiments were conducted with the sensory neurons of different modalities.

Let's consider the reaction of a neuron to the stepwise input influence.

The model of a neuron created by an algorithm and a computer program is granted with the highest preference due to the wide opportunities it provides in manipulating of input signals with the parallel registration of the resulting signals. These advantages, definitely, outweigh the fact that this model can be easily reproduced in the form of an electric device.

The stepwise variation of the input signals influence on the neuron may be simulated by a stepwise variation of $U^+(t)$ (see the diagram in Figure 6).

The character of signal $U^+(t)$ variation will be changed in compliance with the character of the input impacts described in the studied physiological experiments.

For example, in the study of a cold receptor ([8], p.49), the input action corresponds to the curve in Figure 10a. The experiments were undertaken with cold receptors of hamster's muzzle skin.

In the study of mechanoreceptors ([7], p.98), the input action corresponds to the curve in Figure 10c. The experiments were based on the stepwise stretching of the muscle fibers of cancer.

In the analysis of the work of the neuron computer model, the listed types of stepwise input signals were used for the function $U^+(t)$ setting.

The neuron's impulse activity obtained through calculations took the following forms: for evaluating the performance of cold neuro-receptors, see Figure 10b; for evaluating the performance of mechanoreceptors – Figure 10e. In addition, to assess the 'typical' behavior of the sensitive cells receptor in the case of stepwise stimulation, the input signal impact changed according to the example in [9], p.70 - see Figure 10c.

The computed result for a "typical" neuron is presented in Figure 10d.

The metabolism curve of the receptors F_m varying in time by stepwise impact F_{ir} (Figure 11 is borrowed from [9], p.149) coincides qualitatively with the 'typical' behavior of a neuro-receptor when there are similar signals in an input.

The 'silence period' of a neuron corresponds to the latent period.

On the base of comparison of the calculated and the real (taken from the cited literature) output signals, which are caused by identical input signals, the following conclusions can be inferred:

1. The dynamics of change of neuron's impulse activity with the stepwise input impact (as it is described in electrophysiological experiments) coincides qualitatively with the results of computer simulation.

2. When the transitional process of model's adaptation to stepwise input signals is over, the frequency of neuron's output impulses in the model is always half the frequency of synchronization impulses. This combination of impulse frequency at the output of a neuron with synchronizing impulses becomes possible only when there are no signal changes at neuron's entrance (in other words, in the state of a relative rest). It would be justified to assume that the value of synchronizing impulse frequency, which gets to the intermediate neurons, is $2f_a$, where f_a is the frequency of alpha-rhythm observed only in the state of rest and it characterizes intermediate neurons.

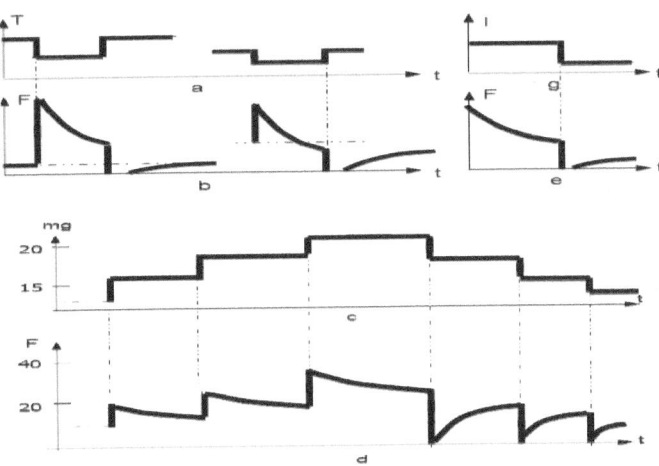

Figure 10: The reaction of a receptor neuron to a stepwise impact

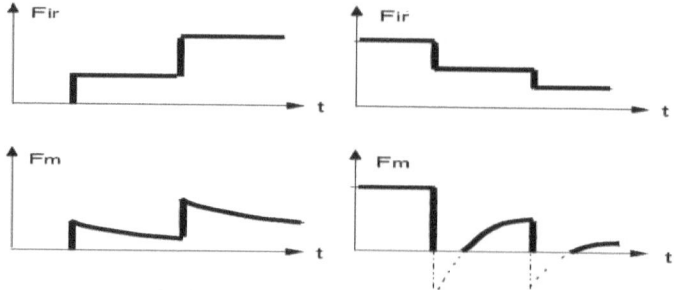

Figure 11: The nature of metabolism in a neuron under a stepwise impact

Conclusion

The author compares the published results of electrophysiological experiments with the responses produced by the computer neuron model at the time when stepwise input signals are imitated.

The qualitative convergence of the frequency changes of neuron's output impulses in electro-physiological and computer experiments stands for the fact that the model corresponds to the live prototype.

The perceptron with two-level memory and time slots of data processing

Using the results of the limbic system analysis, the synthesized model of neuron, and the description of perceptron created by F. Rosenblatt [11], we will construct a model of perceptron with the improved characteristics (comparing to the prototype) which would make the new model to be more similar to its live prototype.

The perceptron may be used in studies of the nervous system as a storage device as well as an information process device. In addition, it can be used in the construction of identifying and learning systems intended for different purposes.

To describe the perceptron as a device used for image recognition would be the most convenient. The block diagram of the perceptron suggested by F. Rosenblatt is presented in Figure 12, where
S - sensor elements, A_i - associative elements, R_j – decision elements, **max** – the unit of maximum selection.

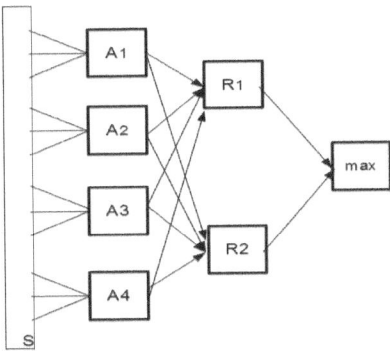

Figure 12: The block diagram of the perceptron suggested by F. Rosenblatt

A recognizable image is projected onto the 'retina', consisting of light-sensitive S-elements. The signals from the S-elements outputs proceed to the inputs of associative A-elements. Each A-element is a linear threshold device. The output signal on its output can be expressed through the threshold function $D(x)$

$$A = D(\Sigma_i(a_i S_i) - \theta) \qquad D(x) = 0, \text{ if } x \leq 0$$

$$D(x) = 1, \text{ if } x > 0$$

$-\infty < a_i < +\infty$ \qquad (a_i – coefficient of relationship)

Signal A can be considered as a secondary feature, which presents an generalized characteristic (comparing to the characteristics the signals of S-elements provide) of the identified image.

The perceptron contains many A-elements which are different in the S-elements they are connected with as well as in the values of the coefficients a_i (relationship) and θ (threshold).

F. Rosenblatt suggested to choose the connection of A-elements with the retina in a random way (with some restrictions). Relating to perceptron as the model of certain parts of the human brain, Rosenblatt supposed that initially, the brain has a random structure and particular connections are formed in the brain only in the result of learning processes.

The outputs of A-elements are connected with the inputs of the decision R-elements. The quantity of R-elements is equal to the number of image classes which are to be distinguished by the perceptron.

The signals of A-elements being multiplied by the weight coefficients λ_{jk}, which characterize the connections between A-elements and R-elements, are summed up.

The output signal of the k-th element R is equal to $R_k = \Sigma_j(\lambda_{jk} A_j)$,
where λ_{jk} - the weight of connection of the j-th A-element with the k-th R-element;
A_j - output signal of the j-th A-element.

The image belongs to the class whose total signal R_k of the corresponding group prevails over the total signals of the other groups.

The training of perceptron is realized by alternate projecting of different images on the retina. For each image, the teacher specifies the class the image belongs to. If the solution found by the perceptron coincides with the teacher's definition, the weights remain unchanged. If the perceptron falsely assigns the image of the k-th class to some other class, the weights of the excited elements in k-th group decrease while the weights in other groups increase.

After quite a long training exercise, a perceptron with random links is able to identify the class of the image correctly. The probability of a correct identification is significantly bigger than the probability of random guessing. This is the case only when the images of one class are excited mainly by R-elements of the same group.

The perceptron could solve even a more complex and practically useful task of image recognition regardless of the image moving throughout the retina if the connection between A-elements and the retina is organized in a particular way.

The perceptron should contain only those sets of A-elements, whose links with the retina are the product of all possible transfers of connection points of any A-element to the retina.

The signals of A-elements can be regarded as some of the secondary characteristics. Each image has a point in the space of these secondary characteristics. Further, we will relate to this space as A-space. The solution the perceptron is obtained by comparing the values of R_k (they are linear in relation to A_j) with each other, i.e. by determining the sign of the difference for each pair of $R_k - R_l$.

As a result, the perceptron performs a linear separation in the space. Therefore, we may state that the perceptron can be trained to solve particular problems of recognition, if the relevant classes of signals are linearly separated in A-space.

The perceptron possesses a remarkable feature to relatively quickly find separating hyper-planes in the training process. The mathematical exploration of the learning process in the perceptron shows that this process is just slightly different from the most advanced of the known methods of laying down a separating hyper-plane which would be the farthest from the points of the two given sets [11].

Although F. Rosenblatt believed that the brain served as the live prototype for his perceptron, his model can be significantly expanded.

It would be interesting to build a perceptron on the neural cells, which were described above. This perceptron would share some properties with the limbic system of the brain, in particular, the property of providing the functional link between the operational and long-term memories. In addition, ring-type neural circuits discovered in the brain structures should be explained in the framework of the described model. The next and the most important issue is to create a synthesized circuit which would preserve the functioning of every intermediate neuron in the processing of multifunctional information.

The named objectives are achieved due to the following facts:

- the work of all neuron's elements is synchronized by a common source of synchronization impulses;
- the processing of sensory information of one modality is always done in the same time slot characterized by specific phase which is defined in relation to the period of synchronization;
- operational information from all sensory inputs circulates in a closed ring with delays related to the number of presentations of initial information on sensor inputs;
- the transfer of information from RAM into the long-term memory is carried out after it has been compared to the information contained in the buffer connected with the long-term memory.

Only that part of information arrives to the output of the block of comparison, which characterizes the difference (the newness of operational information) between the information images.

The resulting block diagram of perceptron is presented in Figure 13; for the block diagram of a buffer in a delay ring line, see Figure 14.

The block diagram of the synthesized device consists of a sync generator (1) connected to the phase ring distributor (2). Each phase output of the ring distributor (2) is connected with a synchronizing input of afferent neurons (3). Sensory inputs of afferent neurons (3) are connected with the receptors (4) of an appropriate modality. Regardless of the modality, the outputs of afferent neurons (5) are connected to all inputs of associative neurons (interneurons) (6).

All outputs of associative neurons (6) are connected with the input of buffer memory of the first delay ring line (7).

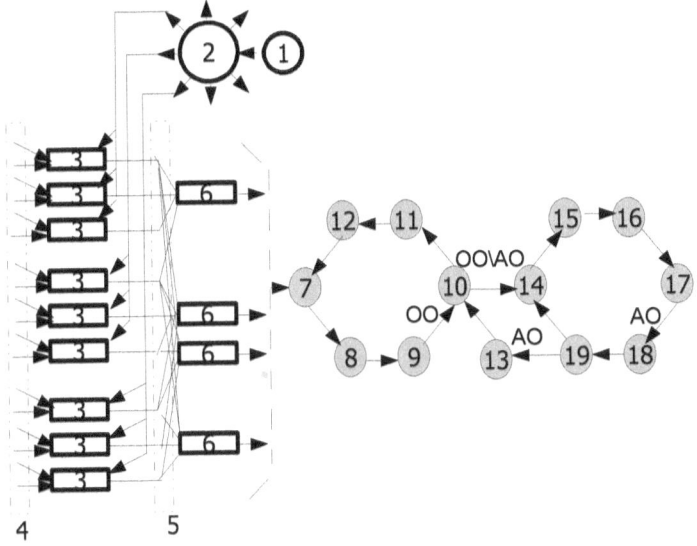

Figure 13: Perceptron

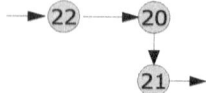

Figure 14: Buffer

The circuit 7-12 consists of the sequentially connected blocks of buffer memory 7-9, the scheme of comparison 10, and the blocks of buffer memory 11-12. Block 10 receives both the operational information from block 9 and the information from the adjacent long-term memory buffer 13. The outputs of block 10 links it with the buffer block 11 of the left ring as well as with the buffer block of the right ring. Blocks 14-19 sequentially connected with each other create the second delay ring line. Block 18, which is connected with blocks 17 and 19, is the block of long-term memory. Block 19 has two outputs, which link it with block 14 and the long-term memory buffer 13. All the units in Figure 13, except for 18, 10, 13, and 19 (they form delay ring lines in the scheme as it was mentioned earlier) might be divided into functionality sub-blocks. This leads to the simplified scheme of Figure 14: unit 20 – the counter of occurrences of the same input information; 21 – the scheme giving permission for the information to be transferred from buffer to buffer along the ring line; 22 – the actual buffer of memory. Blocks 7-9, 11, 12, and 14-17 include the fragment 20-21-22 presented in Figure 14.

Each output of phase ring distributor (2) functions as the source of synchronization impulses for the neuron model presented above.

Let us consider the working process of the mechanism presented in Figure 13. The sync generator (1), which synchronizes the operating of the whole circuit, sends impulses to the ring phase distributor (2). The frequency of the generator is the maximum impulse frequency, which passes through a nerve. For a human, it is about 800 Hertz.

This rate varies from individual to individual and, in the case of one person, it experiences fluctuations which may be caused by numerous reasons. The rhythm defined by impulse generator is considered to be the main biological rhythm of the body. The chapters "Sync generator of the neural network and its live prototype" and "Synchronization in neural networks" suggest more information on the origin of synchronizing.

So, with the help of the ring phase distributor (2), the synchronizing impulses of generator (1) pass (with different phases) to the neurons (3), which process information of different modalities, and synchronize their work.

The above means that during each working cycle of the ring phase distributor (2), the brain by turns (not simultaneously!!!) processes information such as auditory, olfactory, tactile, of thermal receptors, visual blue, visual red, visual yellow, for one eye, for the other eye, from intero-receptors of each modality and so on.

At some point in time, the brain is busy with intellectual work, in the other point in time – using the same neurons, the brain will operate, let's say, the equally important process of urinating. Hence, associative neurons (6) alternately process the sensory information of all modalities in a cyclic way. For this process, as already indicated, the role of a synchronizer is performed by the pulse generator (1), which is connected with the ring phase distributor (2).

The special feature of the ring phase distributor relates to the fact that it has as many outputs as there are phase timing channels (time slots) in the BLS. During a working cycle, the output channels of the distributor (2) get activated in turns. The impulse frequency at each output of the phase distributor f_k is related to the primary biorhythm f_0 and their relationship can be expressed through ratio $f_0=kf_k$ where k is the number of time slots. The phase of impulse series passing through one channel is unique and it differs from the phase of the next time slot by value $1/f_0$. All outputs of afferent neurons, regardless the modality of input signals, are processed in parallel by associative neurons (6). This kind of link is realized to improve the reliability of information processing. In addition, this connection provides the unchanged working of the scheme when the associative neurons, except for one, cease working. In other words, this does not influence the working ability of the brain as a whole (remember Louis Pasteur who successfully worked after a big part of the brain had been resected).

In summary, every associative neuron processes information from all afferent neurons by turns.

Outputs of all associative neurons (6) are connected with block 7, the input block of buffer memory of the first delay ring line. This block performs memorizing of a spatial-time code. Further, for the convenience, this code will be presented by Operative Image (OI).

If inhibitions, corresponding to the OI, are presented to the system several times, this causes the transfer of information from buffer memory (7) to buffer memory (8). After the next several presentations at sensory inputs of inhibitions corresponding to the OI, the memorized information moves from buffer memory (8) to buffer memory (9) and further on along the ring. Therefore, each memory buffer (7, 8, 9, 11, and 12) is provided with a counter (20) of presentations of information (corresponding to OI) as well as with schema (21) giving a permission for the OI to be transferred to the next buffer along the ring line if the number of presentations exceeds the specified constant. Figure 14 shows the block diagram of a buffer memory block (under the unified number (22)) consisting of blocks (20) and (21) described above.

The ring, where the operational information moves, has been discovered morphologically and, in Neurophysiology, it is known as the ring of Papez. Actually, in the limbic system of the brain, which consists of two rings of Papez, the transfer of information from buffer to buffer (in terms of neurophysiology: from core to core) is accompanied by a simultaneous process of information filtering. However, the suggested model is not expected to perform these functions.

In block (7), the OI circulating in the ring gets adjusted by the arriving new information. In block (10), the OI circulating in the first ring of Papez is compared to the Image from the long-term memory (18), which has arrived from the buffer (13). It would be appropriate to relate to the information retrieved from the long-term memory as Archival Image (AI).

Only the information which describes the difference between the corresponding OI and AI (in other words, the newness of OI in relation to AI) is allowed to the output of the schema of comparison (10).

The information characterizing the difference between AI (retrieved from memory (18) and proceeding to blocks 19, 13, and 14) and the current AI, which has been formed in the result of the work of comparison block (10) and block (14), arrives to the input of block (14).

The information corresponding to this difference circulates from block (15) to blocks 16 and 17 and it adjusts AI in the long-term memory (18). The OI circulates from block (7) in the first ring of Papez; due to the corresponding number of presentations, the OI passes blocks (8) and (9) and gets finally to the comparison block (10).

Since the perceptron simulates some functions of the brain limbic system, it is necessary to preserve the parallelism of the structures in the model with the ones in its live prototype. For this purpose, it would be sensible to introduce the list of analogies between the blocks of the perceptron and the formations of the limbic system stated in [1].

LBS structure	Block number in perceptron
The first ring of Papez	
Pontobulbar core of reticular formation	7
Mesencefal core of reticular formation	8
Medial core of septum	9
Fields of hippocampus	10, 14
Lateral nucleus of the septum	11
Hypothalamus	12
The second ring of Papez	
Mammilar cores	15
Frontal (limbic) cores of thalamus	16
Singular section of the limbic cortex	17
Neocortex	18
Entorhinal part of the limbic cortex	19
Dentate fascia	13

Of course, each version of the perceptron as a part of the brain reflects the designer's limited representations of the way how the BLS operates. Therefore, the correction of the above diagram will depend on further bio engineering contemplating of the nature of information processing fulfilled by the brain.

The suggested model of perceptron demonstrates how a part of the brain functions. To confirm the legitimacy of the model, some physiological observations will be discussed below that will provide the arguments for the correctness of the main principles laid into the scheme of the model.

The author holds that some observations of neurophysiologists approve the existing principle that all operational functions in CNS are classified by phase.

According to Livanov, "the synchronization between different parts of the cortex at the theta rhythm frequency and the occurrence of phase coherence between these parts are both of crucial importance for gaining and implementing of the memorized reactions" (page 159 [1], [29]).

"The direct dependence of theta waves in the hippocampus on the rhythmic discharges of septum neurons was revealed by methods of correlation analysis, which showed that discharge of each septum cell occurs with a continuous time relation to a certain phase of theta waves" (page 167 [1]).

"The septum neurons with their rhythmic activity and their ability to influence the entire dendritic pyramid system of hippocampal fields CA_3, supposedly, serve as a synchronizer of the interaction of counter excitation flows. Modulating the state of the dendritic system rhythmically, they may create the conditions when the signals, which arrive at strictly defined discrete intervals of time, are subjected to interaction (comparison)" (page 251 [1]).

Probably, the septum plays the role of a synchronizing device which rhythmically regulates the excitability of the dendritic pyramid system CA_3 and creates such conditions that only the signals coming in certain time micro intervals would be subjected to comparison" (page. 267 [1]).

In 1920, Forbes reported that in the CNS, in addition to open neural circuits, there are complex closed circuits. These self-stimulating closed reverberating circuits possibly create the basis of the short-term memory (page 133 [28]).

In 1957, Eccles assumed that closed reverberating neural circuits are the source of alpha rhythm ([31]).

Since the author does not claim the originality of such functionality schemas as 'producing of a signal reflecting the newness of information', 'transferring of newness', 'receiving information from two different directions', etc., some corresponding references are listed below.

The model of newness filter can be found in [27], pages 165 and 221.

The methods of images comparison are presented in [27], page 142.

The working algorithm of newness detection is discussed in [27], page 158.

Since the biological memory is associative and distributed (the system model of associative memory is described in [27], page 19), the examples of the technical implementation of the recording (or updating) process and reading of long-term information can be found on page 38, [27].

Since each neuron has many inputs and they can receive and process the data coming simultaneously from two (or more) different directions, the process of receiving information from several directions is technically realized already in the model of a single neuron.

Considering the interaction between two layers in the perceptron (see the fragment in Figure 15a) may contribute a lot to a better understanding of the working process of the perceptron. Figure 15b shows the nature of the relationship between the neurons of the first and the second layers in the perceptron.

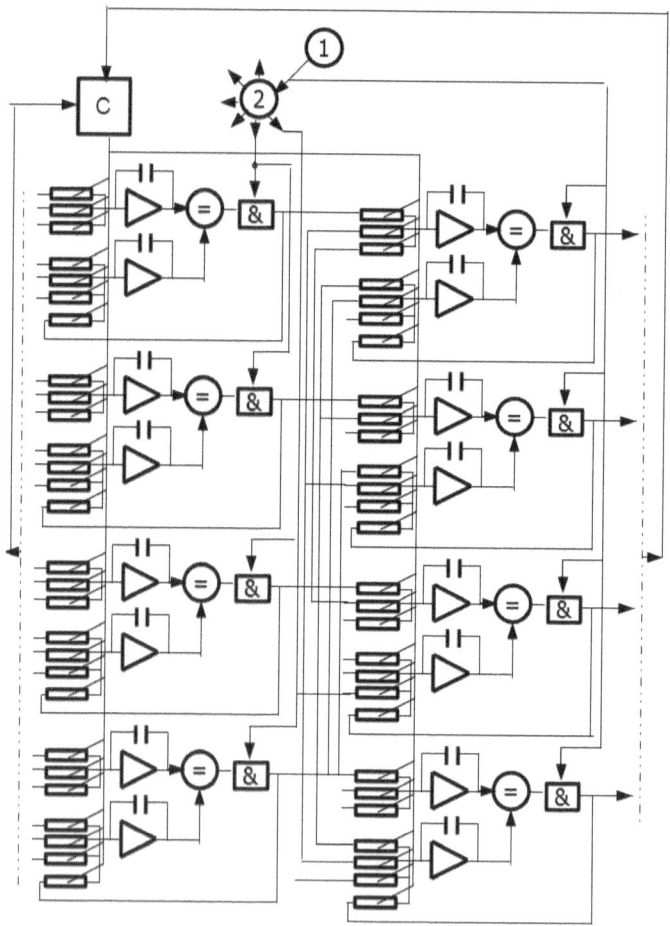

Figure 15A: Perceptron (two layers of neurons)

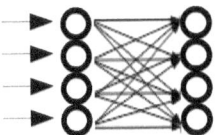

Figure 15b. The nature of relationship between two neighboring layers of neurons

The scheme in Figure 15a is organized as follows:
Sync generator (1) is connected with the ring phase distributor of impulses (2), the control scheme of perceptron's learning (LM), and the inputs of the coincidence blocks of neurons in the second layer (6).

Each output of the ring phase distributor (2) is connected with the coincidence blocks of the first layer neuron groups (3) whose function is to process information of one specific modality.

The output of each neuron of the first layer (3) is connected to the neurons of the second layer in the following way: to the excitatory inputs of about half of the-second-layer neurons and to the inhibitory inputs of the other half of the-second-layer neurons (6).

All the inputs of the first layer neurons (3) and the outputs of the second layer neurons (6) are connected to the control unit of perceptron training (CU) which is associated with varying resistances of inhibiting and exciting inputs of neurons of the both layers (3 and 6).

The working process of the device will be described with reference to Figure 13.

All neurons of the first layer (3), as it was mentioned earlier, are divided into functional groups. Each group specializes in processing information of - one modality type corresponding to its time slot. Obtaining information from all these groups is performed in the moment when output impulses appear at the appropriate output of the ring phase distributor (2).

The work of the neurons of the second layer (6) is also synchronized by a sync generator (1). If the ring phase distributor (2) had had a single phase at the output which had matched impulse phase of the sync generator (1) – (i.e. all neurons in the first layer had been united into a single group by the phase of information processing), the working process of perceptron would barely have differed from the known schemes. The division of information processing by phase in neurons of the first layer (3) allows to get 'decision' in the neurons of the second layer (6) which relate to the classification of images processed by each individual group of neurons in the first layer (3).

In addition, the dynamic impulse pattern at the outputs of neurons of the second layer (6) is able to reflect the 'related' images which appear at the- first-layer neurons' inputs. However, in this case, a more complex mathematical processing of the output is required.

The control unit (CU) performs the iterative calculation of such values of resistance variables at input integrators of neurons of both layers, which would enable the perceptron to correctly classify the Images arriving to its entrance. The role of CU is always fulfilled by a computer program. The algorithm of such a program is described by an iterative process of topology creation of a classifying neural network.

This perceptron learning algorithm is known [26] and used to separate classes of input patterns that would comply with the hypothesis of compactness. The role of a 'teacher' may be performed by a person or by an expensive automatic system with the mechanism of precise recognition.

Conclusion

The perceptron model of recognition, learning and memorizing in the BLS has been discussed. The perceptron built on the neural elements possesses a synchronizing mechanism, which allows to identify the information arriving in different time slots. The synthesized model of learning and memorizing in the BLS is a complementary engineering part for the well-known structure of the BLS.

The author realizes that, during time slots when information from neuro receptors of each modality is processed, the topography of the holographic neural network depends physically on the phase of coherent bio-photons with the help of which the neurons exchange information.

Sync generator of the neural network and its live prototype.

The synchronization rhythm in a live organism is called the main biological rhythm of the body. It would be sensible to discuss the two main hypotheses about the nature of this synchronization.

The first hypothesis is based on the assumption of N.Wiener [11] that the brain has a sort of nonlinear self-oscillating oscillators. Before N.Wiener, it was B.B. Kashinsky who put forward the hypothesis about the oscillatory nature of the structural elements of the nerve tissue [13]). Generally speaking, some known structural elements of the brain may already provide the sync oscillation. The computer experiment held by Aninos (see [2], p. 158) illustrates this. In paper [2], the determined neural network is presented. The structure of its internal connections is determined by the matrix of connection coefficients. The elements of the matrix may take zero or non-zero values depending on the fact whether the connection between individual neurons exists or not.

The non-zero matrix' elements of connection characterize (in compliance with the sign) the connection of one neuron with an exciting or inhibiting input of another neuron. If the connection coefficient between two neurons is zero, there is no synaptic contact between them. The dimension of the matrix of connections, i.e. the number of neural elements of the neural network, is also defined by parameters. The networks are formed by populations of 200-1000 neurons. The dynamics of such a neural network was considered as a Markov process. Every neuron can have three states: rest, excitement, and absolute refractoriness. After the excitation of some neurons, all the neurons which have a synaptic contact with them receive excitatory or inhibitory signals depending on the nature of the existing connection between them. All the incoming signals coming to neuron are algebraically summed up and the sum determines the current level of excitability of the neuron. When the threshold value of the neuron is reached, the neuron itself becomes the source of excitation. If the arrival of the signals coincides with the absolute refractory period of the neuron, the latter does not react to them.

In the computer experiment, the coefficients of the matrix were determined by the generator of random numbers. This defined the topology of the neural network. Aninos analyzed the dynamics of network behavior in time for each version of the network.

"Extensive computer experiments in simulation of the neural network allowed to reveal its clearly expressed ability to create a self-sustaining activity of a cyclic type" [2].

Figure 16 shows the curve of activity of a neural network obtained by counting the total number of excited neurons in time. Each type of cyclic oscillations is determined mainly by the number of inhibitory inputs, the excitation threshold, and the density of inter neuron contacts. The networks of 150 or less neurons were unable to sustain a continuous activity.

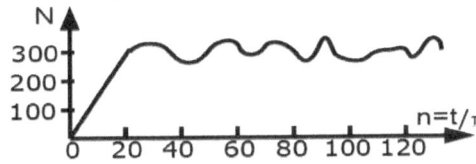

Figure 16: The curve of activity of a neural network.

The ordinate axis N - the number of exciting cells.
The abscissa axis n = t/τ, where
t - duration of the experiment
τ - the synaptic delay of a neuron.

The membrane of nervous cells is the place where a real physical process occurs. Moving randomly, fast electrons get through the membrane. Slowly moving ions diffuse not so fast that leads to accumulating of ions with different charges on the opposite sides of the membrane. This produces an electric field, which forces the electrons to move through the membrane towards the positively charged ions while holes move in the opposite direction.

Numerous carriers are located near the membrane and form such layers, which gradually start preventing further migration of carriers through the membrane until the movement ceases completely. The electrical thickness of this energy gap varies. There always will be one more subtle place. In this place, the electric field can become so strong, that it may cause a short circuit in layers. Since electrons are quickly redistributed, the blocking layer disappears and the accumulated ions freely pass through the 'gate'. The cell takes its original state and, then, everything is repeated.

If electrodes connected to an electrometer are placed on the both sides of the membrane, the electrometer will detect the increase of potential, and, then, a sharp rise - an impulse. A cell generates an impulse at the time determined by its state.

This well-known explanation of the physics on how nerve cells work, helps to design a possible mechanism of the neurons' synchronized working.

The capacity built of energy layers of the membrane is characterized by a certain value of dielectric constant, which, in its turn, depends on the state of the environment.

In the computer experiment with a deterministic network of neurons, which was described above, it was shown that any topology of neural network is characterized by periodic fluctuations (with some restrictions) of its activity. These fluctuations of activity describe the dynamics of exchange processes in the network, produce a dynamic impact on dielectric permeability value of the membrane, and may even synchronize the neurons which are not electrically connected with a reverberating group.

This is one of the possible ways of local communication creation in dynamic systems.

The possible source of synchronization, which is located in the thalamic nuclei, should also be considered [21]. A possible script would be that this oscillator electrically affects blood known as a conductive substance. The impulses can be detected even in the cardio pulse wave (the frequency is about 1000 Hz). It is already a historical fact that regular cardiographs, wherever they are used, have the bandwidth up to 100 Hz. As a result, there never has been a cardiographer which would have registered a high frequency modulation.

The mentioned frequency is special – its value coincides with the detected maximum frequencies in the brain. Within short periods of observation (minutes), this frequency reveals weak fluctuations in a person and it differs from person to person. This frequency defines how fast the incoming information is processed in a body.

Synchronization in neural networks

It is important to note that although in the model of a neuron (Figure 6), the external sync generator is electrically connected to each neuron, in the live prototype, the connections realized in the purpose of synchronization appear to be missing.

Before starting the analysis of the relations between a synchronization source and synchronization objects, some comments about synchronization are to be made.

Synchronization is a form of self-organization. It is defined as a property of various material objects and it produces the single rhythm for co-existence against the background of different individual rhythms and, sometimes, very weak communications (Blekhman [14]).

The first mentioning of self-synchronization of dynamical systems with weak communications goes back to Christian Huygens (1629-1695). He performed an experiment with pendulum clocks [14] and inferred from it that the two pendulum clocks with unsynchronized pace gradually change their pace and come to synchronized working when the both are mounted to the same wall.

Self-synchronization as a feature is not limited to mechanical systems but it is a part of all dynamic systems under certain conditions. The phenomena of synchronization in dynamical systems with weak communications between the elements are mathematically justified in the monograph by Blekhman [14]. This work as well as his other book [15], contains multiple examples of the synchronization phenomenon in biology and medicine.

The so-called weak communications between neurons in the brain can be sustained by conductive blood and lymph. Therefore, direct communications ("wires") between neurons are not required in order to make synchronization possible - it becomes possible due to periodic oscillations in the biochemistry of the environment (for example).

Coherent bio-photons emitted by cells also can be the source of synchronization.
It is an interesting fact that in addition to internal synchronization between neurons, the synchronization can be provided by an external source if its oscillations are close to the frequency of the internal sync generator or a multiple of it.

There was a case when the alpha rhythm was captured by an external disturbance source (flashing lights) with the frequency around 10 Hz ([2], p.92). Even a more intriguing fact is that the capture of alpha rhythm takes place when only the hands of the randomly chosen subjects are exposed to the pulsed light (the subjects do not see the light).

The following experiment also serves as an example of the external synchronization. A metal sheet is mounted parallel to the ceiling and 400 V AC voltage is supplied to it. The floor is grounded. At a frequency of about 10 Hz, a person in the room starts experiencing "definitely unpleasant sensations" [2].

Thus, we can assume that the neurons like all the objects of the material world possess the ability of internal self-synchronization and external synchronization.

Conclusion

The existence of synchronization in all live systems is an indisputable fact.

The period of cyclic activity of perception in time slots

The hypothesis of cyclic activation of perception in time slots for processing data for every neuro receptor modality, implies a micro period of data processing and then, a relatively long pause (its length is equal to the cycle period) during which the same neurons process the data of the other active time slots. Then, the neuron renews processing the data of the observed modality. Since the most experimental data has been collected in the field of visual perception, it would be sensible to apply first the analysis of visual perception mechanism to confirm the proposed hypothesis.

Referring to the factual data, we will try to calculate the period of cyclic working of the vision time slot. The tachy-scopic explorations held in the field of visual objects identification ([13], p.122) will be taken as the basis for further calculations.

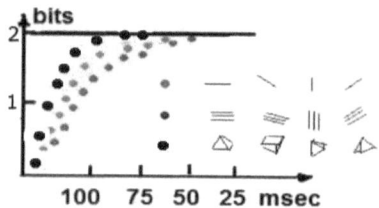

Figure 17: Identified data vs. identification time in the visual identification process.

Figure 17 shows time characteristics of the visual identification process of some geometrical images of different complexity:

The abscissa axis – time of recognition of a visual object in milliseconds.
The ordinate axis - quantity of identified information in bits.

It is important to remember that the time of identification consists of the time of initial processing of visual information and the time required for making the decision. The second time component is difficult to be defined and, probably, it will be considered as a processing error in the final value of the target period of cyclic working of the vision time slot.

The classical problem of Buffon ([19], p.38) is taken as a mathematical basis for the subsequent discussion:

Let a plane be covered with parallel lines with distance 2a between them. A needle with length 2L (L < a) is thrown on the plane at random.

What is the probability that the needle will cross any of the lines while falling (Figure 18)?

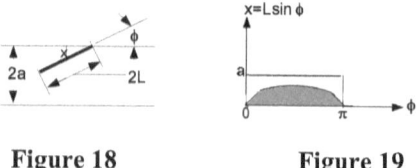

Figure 18 **Figure 19**

Figure 18: Illustration of throwing a needle on the ruled plane in the problem of Buffon
Figure 19: Illustration of the calculation of the geometric probability of crossing a line by a needle.

Denote the distance from the center of the needle to the nearest of the parallel lines through **x**; and the angle created by the needle with the line through **Φ**.
All positions of a dropped needle are totally defined by the points of the rectangle with sides **a** and **π**.

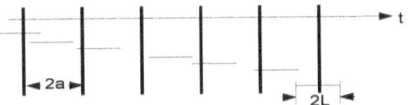

Figure 20: Examples of location of micro periods of visual image identification on the time axis. The vertical bars mark the active periods of the vision time slot.

Figure 20 illustrates that the intersection of the needle with the line becomes possible if the following equation is true:

$$x <= L \sin Φ.$$

According to the above assumptions, the target probability is the ratio of the shaded area (Figure 19) to the area of the rectangle.

$$p = 1/aπ \int_0^π L\sin Φ \, dΦ = 2L/aπ$$

Let us change the conditions of the Buffon problem.
As a "needle", we will use a geometric segment with the length equal to the time of the visual image presentation. We will use the perpendiculars to the horizontal axis of time as parallel lines. The distance between the parallel lines is equal to the length of the desired period of the clock frequency. The thickness of each perpendicular line is equal to a part of the period when visual information processing occurs in a corresponding time slot. Due to the smallness of the ratio between the time slot duration and the sync frequency period, the thickness of perpendicular line is neglected.

In the Buffon problem a needle creates any angle with the closest parallel line, in our case this angle is always equal to 90 degrees. This means that the time slot during which a visual image is exposed to the viewer is always superimposed on the Time axis (see Figure 20). It is assumed that the beginning of this time slot is uniformly distributed in the required period of sync frequency.

In Figure 20, the horizontal segments, which are placed in parallel with Time axis for the demonstration purposes, indicate presentation periods of visual images different in length and the moment of presentation; the vertical bars indicate the activity period of visual perception.

The exposed image can be identified only in the case if the time of its presentation overlaps with the time of the activity of a corresponding time slot. The probability of this event is equal to the probability that a needle will cross one of the parallel lines on the plane. In our case $\Phi = \pi/2$, this probability is

$p = \tau/T$, if $\tau < T$ ($T = 2a$, according to Figure 20)

$p = 1$, if $\tau >= T$

If exposure time increases, the probability of overlapping of this interval with the time slot of visual activity grows proportionally to the value of the exposure time. If the exposure time of a visual object is bigger or equal to the required period between neighboring time slots of visual perception, the probability will be equal to 1.

The accuracy calculation error may stem from the following issues: the time spent on image identification, the variation of the visual time slots within one subject in the course of an experiment, the difference between the visual time slots revealed by different persons, and, finally, from the duration of time slots.

The break point on the curve (see Figure 17) corresponds to the equality of the duration of the visual image presentation and the minimum time length between two neighboring visual time slots.

As shown in Figure 17, this time is equal to 50 milliseconds, i.e. the working frequency of time slot activity is about 20 hertz. Any time slot can be characterized the same way. This value 20 hertz is equal to the duplicate frequency of alpha rhythm.

This finding replicates the results obtained in the simulation of a neuron.

Conclusion.

The problem of Buffon is used to estimate the length of the period between two neighboring visual time slots. This was done on the base of the experimental data collected by the physiologies specializing in vision. The obtained result confirmed the correctness of the assertion that the period of time slot activity is equal to double period of the alpha rhythm.

Identification of time slots

Identification of time slots and their phases of activity is carried out with the purpose to identify the main body systems which are operated in regime of time-sharing. The knowledge of these phases will allow to perform the differential analysis of individual subsystems of the organism. In addition, the assessment of the relationship between such subsystems will also become possible. The phase of any time slot (chosen as the easiest phase for determining) may be taken as a zero phase.

Visual time slots. Instrumental support: sources of coherent light of blue, yellow, and red colors.

The identification method. One eye is completely closed. The experiment is conducted in a dark room. The flashing laser light causes the following reaction: the increased value of impulse frequency is observed in the corresponding time slot; then, the value of impulse frequency gradually declines to approximately 9Hz steady state.

So, presumably, six time slots are engaged into the processing of visual information (three for each eye).

Auditory time slots. Instrumental support: a sound generator, a soundproof room.

The identification method. For each ear (the second is tightly closed with an inserted hearing protector), the sound of frequency $f_0 = df$ with fixed phase is produced in a soundproof room. The auditory time slot, which responds to this frequency, answers with spike activity. The frequency of the pulses gradually falls to about 9Hz in the state of stillness. The same procedure is performed for the frequencies $f_0 + i\, df$ ($i = 0,1,2,.. n$; $df = 1$ Hertz) and for every ear. The frequencies used in the test may be chosen arbitrarily. The expected minimum of the existing auditory time slots is two for each ear, but all audio frequencies are handled, possibly, by more time slots.

The sense of smell. Instrumental support: the hermetically sealed source of smell of a certain modality. One nostril is tightly closed. The source of smell is opened abruptly that activates the corresponding time slots. In this case, the expected response will be similar to the one described above. It would be sensible to run such an experiment with the sources of different odors. It is assumed that there are, at least, two time slots associated with the stereo olfaction by both nostrils.

The perception of taste. The source of taste of a certain modality is placed on the tongue of a subject (after several hours of fasting). The activated time slot is associated with the perception of taste, its reaction time is assumed to be similar to the one described above. It would be reasonable to conduct the experiment with different taste modalities. At least, one time slot is involved into processing of taste information.

The sense of touch. Instrumental support: a mechanical vibrator with controlled frequency of vibration. Tactile stimuli are applied to the index finger of a subject. The corresponding time slot, which is responsible for processing tactile information, is activated. The expected response in time is similar to the one described above. The tactile stimulation of different parts of skin as well as of various acupuncture points is of special interest

Cognitive time slots. In order to identify time slots responsible for processing information related to thinking process, it is recommended to conduct the analysis while the subject is working on intelligence tests. The subject is to be free from the influence by other stimuli. The time slots activated at solving intelligence problems may be reasonably classified as the thinking ones.

The cardiovascular system. Instrumental support: a treadmill. The test is based on a sharp transition from the state of dormancy to the state of active movement, and then – a sudden withdrawal from the movement. It is assumed that the time slots which get activated by the changes in physical activity load are responsible for the operating of the cardiovascular system.

The thermoregulation system. The test is based on the abrupt change of temperature (rise or fall). Such a change can be reached, for example, by fast moving of the subject from room with low temperature into the room with high temperature. The activated time slots are associated with thermoregulation of the body.

Digestion. The test is conducted after several dozens of hours of fasting. The subject is asked to take, for example, some liquid of alkaline or acidic nature by turns. Activating of time slots can be also checked in the subject after taking a medicine for diarrhea, vomiting, etc. The activated time slots are associated with the related functions of operating the processes of digestion and water control.

Breathing. The subject is asked to hold the breath as long as possible. The observations are performed before, during and after the breath holding. It is assumed that the time slots activated during breathing realize operating of the relevant functions of respiration.

The use of hypnosis. It is proved to be efficient to conduct a series of experiments with the subject affected by hypnosis. The advantage of such experiments is the ability of the subject to focus on the performance of a particular function. In addition, some tests are easier to be imagined by the subject than to be technically carried out by the researcher.

It would be also very useful to carry out series of experiments to study the processing of information provided by the vestibular apparatus and, also, some other experiments which would be performed in a recompression chamber.

The author believes that the control loops, which include the neuro receptors responding to certain hormones, do not work in compliance with the scheme described above since the feedback can be carried out at the biochemical level too.

The number and the objectives of the tests to be conducted should not be limited by those recommended above. The exploration of testing methods in order to pick out the ones which would suit to such complex system as the human being is already the subject for a serious study by itself.

The research in daily and seasonal rhythms of time slots could also contribute a lot to the issue.

Conclusion

Some methods how to determine phases of activity of time slots are proposed. The discussed time slots are responsible for processing information of different modalities.

Numerical evaluation of time slot activity (under weak perturbations)

Although the management in a time slot is represented by a binary sequence of impulses, according to the chapter "Delta modulator of the model", it is clear that in increments, this binary sequence represents the analog function, the characteristic of a time slot activity.

Therefore, the clearest way of representing the activity of the time slot would be through the numeric characteristics describing the analog function's "behavior" in time. The analog function (only for weak perturbations) is given in (11) (see chapter 'The BLS in the light of the Automatic Regulation and Control Theory') as

$$\Phi_o(t) = \Sigma_i (\Sigma_j (C_{ij}*t^j))*e^{\lambda_i t}$$

where i=1.. m;
j=0,..,k_j-1;
$\lambda_1, \lambda_2,..., \lambda_m$ - different roots of characteristic equation $D(\lambda) = 0$
$k_1, k_2,.. k_m$ - their multiplicity, then $\Sigma_i k_i = N$

Consequently, the analog function can be characterized by the table with coefficients C_{ij}, λ_i, k_i.

Different pathologies of the time slots will be translated into the quantitative components of the table. These coefficients determine the dynamics of the parameter value fluctuations, which, in their turn, define the activity of the respective time slots. The final judgment of the significance of these coefficients for some pathologies can be made only after some special statistical studies of patients have been performed. For example, when the data has been collected in the study of the representative sample of 'healthy' patients, it is necessary to have the named numeric characteristics of the time slots defined beforehand. These characteristics should correspond to a so-called 'normal' reaction of the time slot studied in a respective test. As a result, it will be possible to determine the values of the boundaries of 'rules', etc.

Conclusion

It is proposed to use parameters of analog function in order to evaluate the activity in time slots. In increments, the analog function corresponds to the binary code produced with the help of the proposed scheme.

Ability to handle EEG.

The modern insight (just please remember that the current work was written in 1984) into the electrical activity of the brain is presented with maximum details in [21]. The work also deserves special attention due to the vast bibliography it suggests. The mentioned paper describes oscillators in the thalamus as the source of synchronizing impulses in the BLS. This fact is important to be used in the analysis of the EEG. The existing devices, which handle and analyze the obtained EEG data, are based on the statistical processing of the signal, which, in its turn, is the algebraic sum of the signals bearing diverse information.

The main EEG harmonics are extracted from the signal by the known devices. The signal is equal to the smoothed algebraic sum of the impulse sequences, which are phase-shifted in relation to each other. These impulse sequences are generated by neurons and they characterize the processing of information of different modalities. When the phase-shifted impulse signals are summed up, some information characterizing the components gets lost; therefore, the value of such summing signal is quite poor.

In the processing of the EEG, it would be reasonable to consider the following points:

1. The electrically conductive blood transfers electrical oscillations throughout all the circulatory system. The frequency of this rhythm is about 1000 Hz and it is the subject for changes with time within one person as well as it varies from person to person. For example, the registration of this rhythm may become possible through the analysis of cardio pulse. It should be noted that a cardiograph traditionally has the bandwidth of 100 Hertz, that is not enough for the task.

2. In parallel, intermediate neurons are involved into the processing of multimodal information, which is performed at random. At a time, the information of only a single modality is processed. Thus, intermediate neurons use time slots for functional separation of multimodal information.

3. The frequency of alpha rhythm is half the value of the frequency of a time slot's cyclic activity.

4. The binary subsequence is actually a record of control function in increments. It is extracted from the output sequence of intermediate neurons and it characterizes each time slot individually.

Taking into account the statements listed above, we can construct the following block diagram of the device. The device detects control functions for each time slot (see Figure 21)

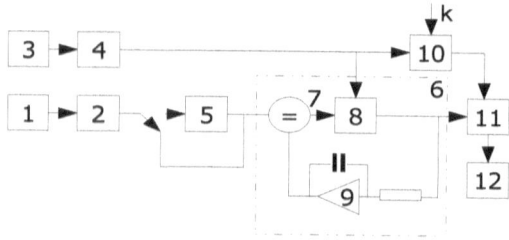

Figure 21: An approximate block diagram of the device for processing EEG data

Figure 21 shows: 1 - EEG sensor, 2 - wide-band amplifier, 3 - sensor of cardio pulse, 4 – band-pass filter for cardio-pulse; 5 - band-pass filter for alpha-rhythm; 6 - delta modulator; 7 - comparison block; 8 - coincidence block; 9 – feedback integrator; 10 - phase-shifting selector; 11 - coincidence block; 12 - recorder.

The working process of the device. From a cardio pulse, which is recorded by the sensor (3) with the help of a band-pass filter with the bandwidth of 200-1000 Hz (4), an impulse signal with the frequency of hundreds of hertz ($\geq$ 600 Hz) is extracted. Further, this impulse signal will be used as a synchronizing one.

The EEG sensor (1) is located above the area of the highest concentration of intermediate neurons. The wide-band amplifier (2) records the analog signal, which is to be decomposed into components.

Delta modulator (6), compiled of a comparison block (7), a coincidence block (8), and an operational amplifier in the mode of integrator (9), is intended for performing the recovery of an impulse signal which would correspond to the analog signal at the delta modulator (6) input.

At a certain stage, the restored binary signal (impulse code) contains all the information on the current state of all neuro receptor inputs – it is processed by intermediate neurons.

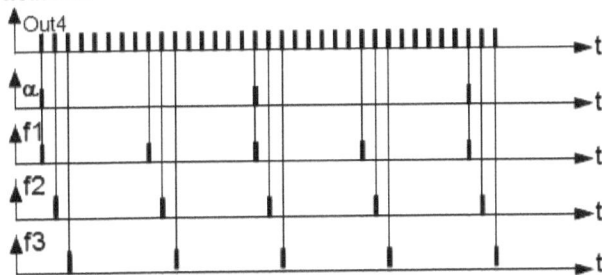

Figure 22: The diagram of the phase shift selector working in time

Within this binary sequence, the phase-shifted sub-sequences of the impulses are located. They characterize the work of the relevant time slots processing neuro-receptors' information of different modalities (see the diagram in Figure 22).

In order to identify all these sequences, the phase shift selector of impulses (10) and the coincidence block (11) are used. Figure 22 may be a good asset in studying the working process of the phase shift selector (10):

Out4 – an impulse sequence from the block (4) output; α - the alpha rhythm, applied to the input of the impulse selector (10); f1 - output impulse sequence emitted by selector (10) when the conditional number of the time slot is equal to 1; f2 - the same when the conditional number of the time slot is equal to 2; f3 - the same when the conditional number of the time slot is equal to 3.

The phase-shift selector (10) shifts the output impulse sequence by the value (k – 1) T, where k is the number of the time slot, T - period of the impulse sequence from the output unit (4). The period of the impulse sequence at the output of the selector (10) is equal to $2/f_a$, where f_a - frequency of alpha rhythm.

The impulses sequence 'cut out' by the phase-shift selector (10) comes to the coincidence block input (11) fulfilling the function of enable signals.

The block of coincidence (11) selects a binary sequence from a series of impulses coming from the output of the delta modulator (6). This binary sequence characterizes the work of the corresponding time slot. Further, the series of impulses, which entered the block of coincidence (11), is directed to the computing device named the recorder (12).

Further representation of binary code, which characterizes the unimodal data processing by intermediate neurons, can be expressed through an analog form for a better clarity. This requires switching from the increment of the binary representation to the analog control function corresponding to its binary original.

With the same recorder (computer) (12), it is possible to numerically evaluate the analog control function.

It is important that this device will enable the researchers to observe how the brain processes information in separate time slots.

Here is an incomplete and tentative list of time slots categorized by modality of the processed information:

Visual time slots:
- blue color perceived by the left eye,
- blue color perceived by the right eye,
- yellow color perceived by the left eye,
- yellow color perceived by the right eye,
- red color perceived by the left eye,
- red color perceived by the right eye.

The sense of smell:
- receptors of the left nostril,
- receptors of the right nostril.

Hearing:
- left ear,
- right ear.

The sense of touch:
- a feeling of pressing.

Temperature balance:
- Management of temperature regulation of the body.

Control of blood pressure.
Control of digestion.
Moving control.

Cognitive time slots.
Blood composition control:
- maintaining the blood sugar level,
- maintaining the level of oxygen in the blood,
- maintaining the level of carbon dioxide in the blood,
- maintaining some level of mineral salts and substances in the blood.

A more detailed list of time slots with the defined pertinent phases may be issued only after the physiological experiments with the use of devices similar to the one discussed here will have been done.

The presented method of processing EEG has some limitations due to both the 'noises' in the signal and the low-frequency distortions produced by the tissues of a skull.

If the numerical estimation of these distortions was obtained, the signal could be restored (see Figure 21: block 5 is designed for this purpose).

Conclusion

A new approach to handling EEG data is put forward. This approach is designed to evaluate the time slots activity in relation to information processing carried out by the brain.

The placement of the EEG electrodes

Since the analysis focuses on the BLS activity, the points where the individual fragments of the BLS are projected to (including the acupuncture points) seem to be the most appropriate place(s) where the electrodes measuring the electrical activity of the brain are to be applied.

These points are listed in accordance with [25], p.46. The marking of the points uses the mnemonics of [25]: GB20 – sympatheticus (p.47); 10aMA – vagus; Bl10 – medulla; GB4 - thalamus (p.73); Bl9 – pons; GB7 – diencephalon; GB17 - reticular formation; GB12 - pituitary gland; 3E20 - hypothalamus (p.45).

It would be preferable to assess the activity of intermediate neurons by measuring the signal primarily in points GB17 (a reticular formation, the top), 3E20 (the hypothalamus, the temple), and Bl10 (the medulla oblongata, the nape of the neck).

The functions of these points are known [25] as well as their topography – this explains the above choice of these points.

By processing the information from all exterior and inter receptors of the body, the reticular formation participates in the maintaining of homeostasis state, which always depends on the current needs of the organism.

The hypothalamus is responsible for numerous processes in the human body such as thermoregulation, sleep, fat and water metabolism, sexual function, sweat secretion, etc.

The medulla oblongata is responsible for breathing control, blood circulation, vomiting, swallowing, sneezing, etc.

The topographic anatomy of these and many other points is described in all acupuncture manuals (for example, see [26]). In addition, manuals usually suggest pictures clarifying the location of these points on the skin in different projections and their schematic position in relation to the bones of the skull that facilitates determining of the points' location.

Conclusion

Referring to the known relations between acupuncture points and the corresponding internal structures of the brain, a group of points for EEG analysis has been proposed. The analysis is aimed at splitting of the signal into informational components. The list of the suggested points for the EEG analysis, of course, remains open for further updates.

Analysis of impulse activity of acupuncture points

To start analyzing encephalograms by the method described above, it is necessary, first, to solve the problem of distinguishing between the time slots signals in the situation when input signals are not particularly 'clean' (during an EEG test, signals bearing information of different types may overlap). Besides, the distortions of a signal caused by the skull tissues have never been evaluated either analytically or numerically.

Therefore, in the analysis of encephalograms, the first priority should be given to the analysis aimed at separating the time slots impulse activity which is read from the needles inserted into acupuncture points.

The solution to the problem of distinguishing between the useful signal and the noise (artifacts, mio-electrical activity) is facilitated by the fact that time slots are activated turn-by-turn in time. Distinguishing between the time slots can be performed at the programming level rather than in a scheme.

In order to facilitate the computer recording and processing of the signals read in acupuncture points, we assume that the impulses' duration in acupuncture points is short comparing to the length of activity period of all time slots (sync frequency period) and, therefore, it can be neglected.

Then, the presence of an impulse taken in the j-th acupuncture point at time t can be expressed through the equation $f_j(t) = 1$.

The fact of missing impulse in the j-th acupuncture measurement point at time t can be written as $f_j(t) = 0$ where $f_j(t)$ is a binary function showing the impulse activity in acupuncture point.

Practically, this means that the functioning of an acupuncture point may be encoded as a bit string, the length of which corresponds to the observation time as well as to the synchronization frequency.

It is assumed that certain acupuncture points "service" certain time slots. In other words, the following statements are true.

Statement 1. Let N – a set of acupuncture points. Then, there are its subsets for which the assertion $(f_j(t) = 1)$ & $(f_l(t) = 1) \sim 0$ is true for each t.
If the conditions $j \in W_i$ $(W_i \in N)$ and $l \in W_r$ $(W_r \in N)$ are true,
then $W_i \wedge W_r = L$, where L is an empty set.

Hence, the acupuncture points can be grouped in such a way that the impulses of the points of one group will never coincide in time with the points' impulses of any other group. However, within one group, the impulses of different points may coincide in time.

Statement 2. The equation $f_j(t) = 1$ will be true for any acupuncture point and time t, only if (but not enough)

$$t \in t_{syn} \text{ is true when } j \in W_i$$

where t_{syn} - time appearance of the clock impulse.

Thus, we see that the impulses in each acupuncture point can appear only in certain moments, which coincide with the phase of synchronizing impulses of the corresponding time slot. The phenomenon of synchronization is global in the body and the oscillations take place simultaneously all over the body. Another issue taken into account is that being stimulated by a needle, at the beginning, an acupuncture point turns into an impulse generator. An additional research is required to define the time of adaptation to the irritation, after which the impulse fluctuations become informational in terms of the analysis of the corresponding time slot activity.

The impulse activity of acupuncture points can be used as an additional informational input for the analysis of the psycho-physiological state of a person. But first of all, all acupuncture points are to be classified per time slots. It would be interesting to compare the resulting classification to the one used in the Oriental Medicine.

Conclusion

It is assumed that the analysis of impulse activity of the acupuncture points based on the method of observing changes of the analog function in increments will help to estimate the state of various systems of the body. The analog function will be presented as the binary code, which will characterize the activity of every time slot.

Perceptron and physiological experiments

Once again, let us consider the perceptron presented in chapter ' The perceptron with two-level memory and time slots of data processing '. If the same visual image appears with frequency $2f_\alpha$ (f_α - the frequency of alpha rhythm), the newness of this image will be recorded into the long-term memory of the brain only after its corresponding image will have passed through all the blocks of Papez circuits. An image can make a full way through all the blocks of Papez circuits only if it is exposed 10-13 times for a person (this is also true for cats). The entire process of recording into the long-term memory is carried out on a subconscious level.

Thus, the human beings possess the mechanism of accelerated perception of any information represented in visual images. Taking also into consideration that 90% of the information absorbed by the brain is perceived through the optic tract, it is correct to state that the information presented in visual images is the most efficient for remembering.

Having performed numerous experiments, some American advertising companies drew a conclusion that if an image presented in words, for example, "the smell of hay", shows up for a moment between the frames of a usual film (the author holds that such a moment should last not less than 1-2 milliseconds), it affects the audience. The image is to appear repeatedly, about ten times - the audience definitely does not read the message consciously. Nevertheless, after the movie, the survey respondents mentioned they smelled hay though did not notice any cut-ins while watching.

Even a more interesting example, which supports the concept of *perception*, relates to the accelerated way of teaching people. Works [32] and [33] describe an automated system designed to assist in learning and knowledge control.

In this system, one type of training sessions is based on the principle of supplying learning material in the rhythm of biological processes of the learner. The studied information is offered to the learner in a synchronized way with one of the major biorhythms of the learner, for example, with breathing rhythm, heartbeat or brain (bio) currents. The highest synchronization frequency is equal to the alpha rhythm frequency in this system.

When the proposed system is used for accelerated learning of a foreign language (e.g. English, German or French) without an instructor, it enables the person to learn 3,000-4,000 words (as a passive vocabulary) for 10-12 days, in average, during 80-100 hours of study. When Japanese is the object of study, the passive vocabulary of 1000-1200 hieroglyphs is mastered in the result of 15-20 days of training. When the automated system is used for training people in speed reading, the speed of reading gets doubled after 2-3 days of practicing (the quality of learning is preserved).

In the typing course run by the automated system, the typing speed of 140-170 symbols per minute is gained, in average, within 3-4 days of training.

In the course of autogenic training, the skills of auto training are mastered within 2-4 days of training when the automated system is used.

A course of theoretical and humanitarian disciplines (for example, the Theory of Probability, the Social Psychology or the Line Drawing), which is equal to a university course of one semester, can be studied with grade "Good" within 2-4 days if the automated system is involved into the learning process.

The empirically defined rate of the teaching material presentation, which should be equal to the frequency of alpha rhythm (f_a), is sufficient for subconscious perception. This does not conflict with the assertion that perception occurs already at the frequency twice as high.

Thus, the results obtained in the experiments performed with the use of the synthesized model justify the possibility of increasing the feed rate for learning material twice as fast in the systems practicing a so-called suggestopedia teaching method. As a result, the time required for mastering the material decreases significantly.

The fact of distinguishing between impulses (produced by acupuncture points) by phase and their frequency range could serve as another confirmation of the correctness of the BLS functioning operational model. The well-known classification of acupuncture points was formed thousands of years ago. We may expect the existence of the common phase of impulses for various acupuncture points within every functional group.

If this is the case, then, the relations between functional systems (known in the Oriental Medicine) may be projected on the relations between the operating functions, which realize themselves through different time slots of the BLS.

The frequency of impulses read on the acupuncture points by electrodes stay in the range $[0-2f_a]$, i.e. 0-20 Hz (see [35]), that is the confirmed fact.

It should be taken into consideration that the topography of an acupuncture point influences the phase of its impulses.

At the same time, if the frequency of impulses is defined by the use of a needle inserted into an acupuncture point (the needle is insulated except for its tip whose size is just 20-50 microns), the dynamics of the frequency gets into the range of 0.5-400 Hz [34]. This means that the impulses of neuro receptors located in the area of the studied acupuncture point are superposed on the frequency of $2f_a$. The impulses are caused due to the mechanical irritation the needle produces.

Conclusion

In this chapter, the well-known physiological experiments are considered. These experiments confirm the adequacy of the teaching mechanism to the perceptron model of the brain limbic system.

The chapter suggests the reasoning for the possibility of increasing the feed rate for learning material twice as fast in the systems practicing a so-called suggestopedia teaching method. As a result, the time required for mastering the material decreases significantly.

The General Conclusions

Based on the published descriptions of the morphological and functional structures of the limbic system of the brain, the model of learning and memory in the BLS is synthesized in the form of a self-adjusting phase-impulse system of regulation and control.

The qualitative analysis of the model functioning has been performed, the analytic functions describing the change of the parameters of homeostasis in time have been derived for minor impacts.

The electric model of a nerve cell as the basic building block of the BLS was synthesized. This model complies with the conditions of the functioning of the BLS as a whole. The informational qualitative analysis of functioning of the nerve cell model has been carried out.

The model of the perceptron with the two-level memory and time slots as the instruments of information processing was synthesized. The model is presented as a neural network built of the synthesized elements.

The concept of *time slot* has been introduced. A time slot is a time interval when the information, which has been received from neuro receptors of a particular modality, get processed.
This interval associates with a certain phase of synchronization frequency.

The synthesized model uses the notion of real time sharing between different functions of the BLS that is realized on the same neuron groups.

At the same time, the work of homeostasis control circuit containing various neuro receptors, which are responsive to a variety of hormones, does not fit in the proposed scheme, because the biochemical regulation exists along with the impulse control systems.

The functioning of the synthesized models has been analyzed against their live prototypes. The adequacy of the both was found evident.

The phase and frequency characteristics of impulse activity in each time slot were validated.

The impulse activity of acupuncture points was considered from the viewpoint of functioning of the model as a whole.

The work contains recommendations of the experiments which may contribute a lot to the subject of the study, for example, accelerated learning, EEG analysis, analysis of impulse sequence read from acupuncture points, the identification of time slots in the BLS and so on.

The Afterword

This work was issued as a report in 1983. Now, in 2015, I would like to add to it some points.

It is a well-known fact that there is a system of transmitting information from one cell to another by the means of bio photons (their wave length is 420-720 nm); the bio photons are coherent ([39], [40]). Referring to the holographic nature of memory possessed by the living neural network, it is logical to assume that a particular phase, which characterizes the coherence, activates such configuration inside the complete neural network which corresponds to the processing of sensory information connected to this particular phase. If at the next moment, the coherence of bio photons gets characterized by a different value of the phase, then, the holographic memory will activate the new configuration of the neural network (inside the whole neural network), which will provide the processing of information for the changed value of the phase. This mechanism works for all activated time slots, which have the related phase within the period of synchronization. This approach clarifies how the same neuron structures take part in the solving of different problems. Evidently, the brain is provided with the mechanism of phase distribution. The closed neuron chains (the reverberating chains) found in the brain, can perfectly serve as phase distributors though it is not excluded that the nature invented something more ingenious than this.

Reference

1. О.С.Виноградова. Гиппокамп и память. М. "Наука". 1975.
2. Бионика. Под ред. Л.В.Решодько. Киев "Вища школа". 1978.
3. Методологические вопросы теоретической медицины. Сборник статей. Л. "Медицина". 1975.
4. М.Арбиб. Метафорический мозг. М. "Мир". 1976.
5. Биологические аспекты кибернетики. Сборник работ. М.1962
6. В.Л. Кузьменко и др. Устройство для моделирования нейрона. Авторское свидетельство СССР номер 902033. Класс G06 G7/60, 1980.
7. Г.Тамар. Основы сенсорной физиологии. М."Мир".1976.
8. Физиология сенсорных систем. Под ред. П.К.Анохина.Часть 2. Л."Наука".1972.
9. В.Д.Кейдель. Физиология органов чувств. М."Медицина".1975.
10. К.Прибрам. Язык мозга. М."Прогресс". 1975.
11. Н.Винер. Кибернетика и общество. ИЛ М.1958.
12. Н.Винер. Новые главы кибернетики. "Советское Радио".М.1963.
13. Б.Б.Кажинский. Передача мыслей. М.1923.
14. И.И.Блехман. Синхронизация динамических систем. М."Наука".1971.
15. И.И.Блехман. Синхронизация в природе и технике. М."Наука".1981.
16. В.Чуев, В. Ромашин. Цветовые эффекты на экране чернобелого кинескопа. Ж."Радио", 1973 , номер 8.
17. В.Д. Глезер. Механизмы опознания зрительных образов. М."Наука". 1966.
18. Ю.П.Гоголицын, Ю.Д. Кропотов. Исследование частоты разрядов нейронов мозга человека. Л. "Медицина".1982.
19. В.В.Гнеденко. Курс теории вероятностей. М."Наука".1969.
20. В.Левин. Ускорить неускоряемое. Ж. "Изобретатель и рационализатор", 1982, номер 10.
21. С.М.Осовец и др. Электрическая активность мозга. Механизмы и интерпретация. Ж. "Успехи физических наук", 1983, сентябрь.
22. Микрокомпьютерные медицинские системы. Под ред. У.Томкинса. М."Мир".1983
23. Г.Корн и Т.Корн. Справочник по математике для научных работников и инженеров. М."Наука".1974
24. Частная физиология нервной системы. Руководство по физиологии. Под ред. П.Г.Костюка и Н.П.Бехтеревой.Л."Наука".1983
25. R.Voll. Topographische Lage der Messpunkte der Electroakupunctur. Textband 1.Uelzen.1976.
26. С.В.Свечников,А.М.Шквар. Нейротеехнические системы обработки информации. Киев, "Наукова думка", 1983.
27. Т.Кохонен. Ассоциативная память. М."Мир".1980.
28. Д.Адам. Восприятие, сознание, память. М."Мир".1983.
29. М.Н.Ливанов. Пространственная организация процессов головного мозга. М."Наука".1972.

30. Н.П.Бехтерева. Функциональная характеристика височных лимбических структур у человека. М. "Наука",1971.
31. Дж. Хэссет. Введение в психофизиологию. М."Мир".1981.
32. В.В.Петрусинский и др. Автоматизированная система для обучения и контроля знаний. Авт. свид. СССР номер 635508 от 30.11.1978.
33. Э.Диамент и др. Устройство для обучения. Авт. свид. СССР номер 743007 от 23.06.1980.
34. А.Т.Качан,Н.Н.Богданов. Электрофизиологические особенности точек акупунктуры. Стр. 112-119 в книге "Оптимизация воздействий в физиотерапии". Минск."Беларусь".1980.
35. Н.М.Зуфрин и др. Инфранизкочастотные сигналы точек акупунктуры. В книге "Проблемы метрологического обеспечения измерения параметров случайных полей и сигналов биологических объектов. М.1982. Материалы конференции.
36. Е.В.Айзенберг,Г.П.Комаров,Е.Н.Гак. К вопросу о кибернетических аспектах управления механизмами адаптации в живых системах. В сборнике "Кибернетические аспекты адаптации системы "человек-среда" (тезисы семинара). Под ред. Р.М. Баевского. М.1975. Научный совет по комплексной проблеме "Кибернетика" АН СССР.
37. Е.В.Айзенберг. Распознавание квазипериодических временных рядов. Депонированная рукопись, Номер 2261 пр-Д83 от 21.11.1983. М."ЦНИИ информации и технико-экономических исследований приборостроения, средств автоматизации и систем управления.
38. Е.В.Айзенберг,Ю.А.Смирнов. Модель нейрона. Авт. свид. СССР номер 1084829 от 24.05.1982.
39. http://www.faim.org/energymedicine/measurement-human-biofield.html
40. Meyers, Bryant A. (2013-08-19). PEMF - The Fifth Element of Health

Real-time in Brain Limbic System (short description)

Abstract

Real-time in Brain Limbic System. Every sensor modality is periodically active only at fixed time intervals. Phase distribution between various sensor modalities – concurrent for time-sharing in limbic system. Processing of the period of cyclic activity of 'phase channel'. Electrical model of neuron. Desynchronization can be remarkable in beginning stages of the disease before the body has full results of this desynchronization.

Russian people say about someone who has an unclear mind: "He has phase shift in the brain". This article illustrates an existing scientific basis of this sentence relating to everyone.

The Brain Limbic System (BLS) acts a phase distribution inside the cyclic activity periods of BLS. The phase distribution serves time-separate processing of signals from various sensor systems. The important property of the Brain Limbic System (BLS) is the integral possibility to receive information from reticular formation – the input station for sensor-neurons of various modalities, corresponds with all the fluctuation in the external and internal environment. All external sensor neurons connected to the reticular formation react to sound, light, temperature, pressure, humidity and chemical components of the air etc. In the hypothalamus (an important knot of BLS) specific neurons exist which are sensitive to fluctuation of the body's internal environment. The BLS is responsible for adaptation efforts that bring the homeostasis in a regular condition suitable to changing external conditions and optimal comfort for body functioning.

The following methods are usual for BLS functional activity research: analyzing of behavior response of the BLS by corruption of various of its structures, research of influence on BLS due to electrical and/or chemical stimulation, research of electric activity of separate structures BLS during various behavioral actions, analyzing of neurons impulse activity in separate structures of BLS depending on exterior signals of various modality. The last method is more attractive for engineering access and comprehension.

Short explanations of the experiments:

1. Thin needle-electrodes were implanted into various points of main knots of a cat's BLS (boxes on the Figure 1) and connected to a registration unit;

2. An external irritation was used by short signals (the length near to the neuron impulse length) of light impulses, blinking in various time sequences;

3. A separate experiment was carried out with sound impulses of various lengths, strengths and intervals. In both cases the response was neuron impulse sequences in various "stations" of BLS. The structure of BLS [1] – the object of the research is illustrated in Figure 1.

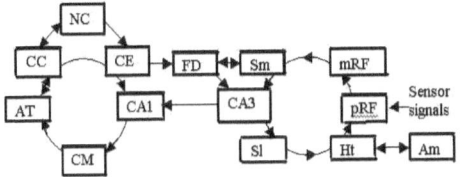

Figure 1. Outline of BLS structure

CA_1, CA_3 hippocampus fields; FD – denticulate fascia; Sm, Sl – medial and lateral septum nucleus; mRF, pRF – mesencephal and pontobulbar parts of reticular formation; Ht – hypothalamus; Am – amigdala; CM – mammilary corpora; AT – frontal limbic nucleus of the thalamus; CC, CE singular and entorhinal parts of limbic cortex; NC – neocortex.

It is interesting to note this drawing from an engineering point of view. The multidisciplinary aspect of scientific brain research makes it impossible to explain brain function using only one profession-related terminology, and I must use a free superposition of engineering terminus on the neuro-psychological territory.

Definitions: Irritation - a sequence of blinking light impulses. Image - a space-time impulse sequence - the response of some Irritation (relevant to each box on the figure). New Image– an opposed to old (from archive) current Image.

Short explanation of observations in [1]. The role of the long storage memory has played the box NC (PC analogy - hard disk). The operative memory displaces in two Papez rings. The right ring services all of the external and internal images. Since the internal Image is constant during the experiment, it is possible to omit the influence. The new Image penetrates internal rings through the pRF-box. The movement from box to box is possible only after some repetition of the same external Image. When the Irritation stops, the Image disappears (not immediately). When the external Irritation changes its character, the movement from box to box continues after a delay of some (2-3) repetitions of new Irritations. The box CA_3 is a comparator. The objects for comparison are the current Image from box Sm and the archived Image from box FD. FD is connected with memory for news (left Papez ring) and 'hard disk' NC. The box CA_3 is not a simple binary comparator: after comparing the current Image from Sm with an archived Image from buffer FD, the News will be moved to the box CA_1.

Important observation: the comparison of one modality Image is periodically active only at fixed time intervals.

The Left Papez ring is a place for circulation of News. The end of processing the News will be written from box CC onto the hard disk NC. From this moment, the comparator CA_3 compares current Images with new archive Images. It is necessary to say, that every Image or Image News moving from box to box becomes some correction by the way. "Target of every transformation in living system is to diminish abundant information" [8].

After analyzing all of the output impulse sequences and comparing them with input signals the conclusions (omitting certain details) are:

1) The impulses in LBS have a standard form (amplitude, length). The coding depend only from the fact "exist or not exist" the impulse in specific time. If the impulse (or impulses) are absent, the delay is multiple to the one impulse length.

Comment: 1) It is typical phase-impulse coding in terminus of technical systems

2) Processing of sensor information is doing in specific phase relatively to some leader frequency.

3) The response on the stimulation is acting regularly during the short period with interval equal to the period of synchronization

4) All impulse sequences are synchronized by some leader frequency.

Comment: the synchronization takes a place yet on the neurons level, see "Model of neuron" [2].

5) Sensor signals of various modalities beginning from the reticular formation have the same trace in the BLS.

Comment: last fact can be better understandable if there exists a time's sharing in the processing signals from various sensor systems. It possible to say that exists phase distribution between various sensor modalities – concurrent for time-sharing in BLS.

For example, we do not hear and see exactly at the same moment (phase shift). The left eye and the right eye do not see exactly at the same time, and so on.

6) For functionality of this system it is necessary for the installation of a pacemaker and phase distributor

7) In our experiments an Image is a topographic distribution of impulse response on external light blinking irritation. But in general cases, an Image includes all possible irritations corresponding to homeostasis control. It is possible to create a specific Image with the help of an acupuncture needle. After 12-13 repetitions the created Image will be loaded into memory (Subcortex). If the choice of acupuncture points is correct, the body has updated rules for best control of homeostasis. It is the explanation of influence through the acupuncture points as a method of correction of BLS transform function.

Figure 2 illustrates a similar correction of transfer function in the technical system of impulse control with feedback. In such systems, the coding of the control signal is based on the modulation of frequency or phase of circulating in the system impulse sequence. The correction of the transform function in similar systems is realized with the help of a correcting chain (- - -).

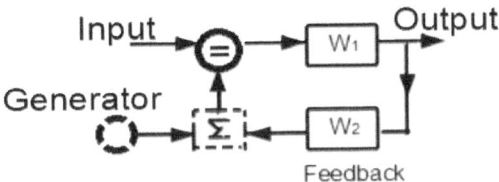

Figure 2. Correction of transfer function in impulse control systems

It is necessary to change the transforming function of the system without touching the W1 box, we need to add some new boxes: Generator of impulses and Summation.

It is simple to see that the transforms functions of the system before correction and after correction are not the same.

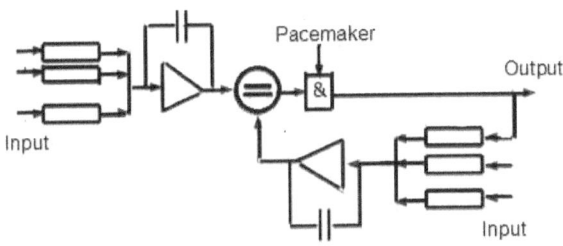

Figure 3. Electrical model of neuron

Comment. The neuron's models [2] can be satisfied to the demands of LBS and shown on [2] Figure 3.

In the Figure 3: box '&' - schema 'AND', comparator in the ring, and two integrators. The comparator sends to its own output the impulse when the value of the output signal of the left integrator overcomes the value of the output signal of the right integrator. The external pacemaker (particularly the impulse generator) is not part of the model, but the moment of the output impulse of the neuron, corresponded to the time of the pacemaker impulse. All resistances in integrators play the role of learning coefficients in the neuron. All neurons are different only by value of learning coefficients. Sensor neurons, neurons for muscles control, neurons for glands controls build a separate group.

The response of the theoretical simulation model of neuron provide the same output results as by various kinds of similar stimulations of the theoretical and real neurons in various experiments. For example, research of neuron receptors of the skin in mouse muzzle, sensitive to cold in [5], research of mechanoreceptors in [6], researches of the neurons in [7].

Analyzing of functioning of the neuron model give the following results:
1) The neuron's model behavior confirms all known (by authors) experiments with living neurons in the similar conditions.

2) In the case of constant input signal the value of output impulse frequency will be equal to half of the pacemaker frequency.

Comment. In another words, the synchronizing frequency in every 'phase channel' equal to the duplicate frequency of a-rhythm, because this rhythm is shown only in quietness state (analog of constant level of irritation). The numbers of 'phase channels' in a living system equal the maximal observed frequency in the brain divided on the duplicate frequency value of a-rhythm. The maximal frequency in the brain less than 900 hertz – the number of 'phase channels' is less than 45 channels. In time all this data systems will be known. Now I can give an outline of the list of control channels.

Synchronized Brain

B.B.Kazhinsky [9] may be the first to write about the existence of synchronization in the brain, Norbert Wiener [10] supposed nonlinear auto-oscillators exist in the brain. About existing closed chains of neurons is written in [11]. Mr. Eccles supposes, that reverberation neurons chains are a responsible for a-rhythm creation. [12]

Comment. For impulse generator creation, it is enough to have two neurons in a closed chain, but to have a connection from one pacemaker to all the billions of neurons seems abundant, and in nature there exists a synchronization of dynamic systems with weak communications without a pacemaker as separate unit. The best mathematical ground for such systems in practice and in high nature is shown by I.I.Blechman [14, 15]. A simple example: two wand watches with pendulum are synchronized on the same wand not depending from the start pendulum's positions.

As in technical systems, living dynamic systems can be synchronized from external synchronizer in the specific limits. For example, when blinking light has a frequency near to a -rhythm, the a-rhythm slightly changes his value and will be equal to the frequency of external synchronizer. In technique exists a special slang for this – 'a capture of frequency'. I am not sure, it seems to me, I have read about this experiment in the book of Walter Grey [16].

The running discrete slides of cinema is a good illustration for existing visual phase channel and external synchronization with help of visual cadre sequence.

Processing of the period of cyclic activity of 'phase channel'

The hypothesis of an existence of cyclic activating phase channels for every sensor modality supposes a short time of activity of every channel during the cycle and than relative long pause of length equal to the cycle period. It is easier to analyze first of all the vision phase channel.

The experimental base for the search is real information – tachyscopic registration of the recognition time for various visual objects [13]. See the draw on Figure 4.

The vertical axes shows a quantity of recognized information in bits, the horizontal axe - time for recognition of visual object in mille second.

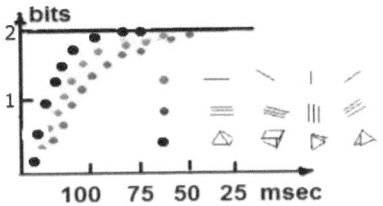

Figure 4. Recognition of visual objects

It is necessary to remember, that the time of recognition includes the time for processing of visual information and time for decisions making. The last component is difficult for separate evaluation. This component will be a ground part of processing error.

Let t - time of observation; T – value of the period, including cyclic activity of all phase channels; p - value of probability of intersection time of observation (t) and moments of activity phase channel for processing of vision information

p = 1, if t >= T (case of 100% recognition)

p = t /T, if t < T

The curve of the probability of intersection time of observation and moments of activity phase channel for processing of vision information will be broken in the point of overcoming to value 1. If we return to the picture 4, we will see, that a crack (for simple recognition) is found by frequency of about 20 hertz (period equal 50 msec). It is the time between every two mini-intervals of channel activity. This value 20 hertz is equal to the duplicate frequency of a -rhythm. This result repeats the results of neuron model searching.

Diseases from the new point of view

When we image the living body as a space-timing system with phase-impulse control located in a "black box", there are a lot of diseases or disturbances we can define in terms of synchronization misbalance, or mixture of 'phases channels'. Examples of desynchronizes (we are not speaking now about biochemical comments for each abnormality):

The known situations when somebody fills various tones of sound as various colors, and visa-versa.

· Various visual, hearing, tactile, and smelling hallucinations as result a 'phases channels' mixture

· Dalton's disease – phase replacing in processing separate colors

· Epilepsy

· Cancer – desynchronized creation of new cells (out of time when it is necessary). And so on.

Desynchronization can be remarkable in beginning stages of the disease before the body has full results of this desynchronization.

References (in **Russian**)

1. Winogradova O.S. Hippocampus and memory. Edition. Science, 1975. Moscow
2. Eisenberg E.W., Smirnoff-Shuff J.A.. Simulation model of neuron. Patent of the USSR № 1084829
3. Blechman I.I. The synchronization of dynamic system. Science, 1971. Moscow
4. Blechman I.I. The synchronization in the nature and technique. Science, 1981. Moscow
5. The physiology of sensor systems (edition by P.K.Anochin). Part 2. Science, 1972. Leningrad .
6. The physiology of sensor systems (edition by P.K.Anochin). Part 2. Science, 1972. Leningrad.
7. Keidel W.D. The physiology of sensor organs. M. Medicina, 1975 (translation from German)
8. Methodological aspects of theoretical medicine (Article of Gelfand I.M., Cetlin M.L.). Medicine, Leningrad, 1976
9. Kazhinsky B.B. The transmission of the thoughts. Moscow 1923.
10. Wiener N. Cybernetics and society. Foreign Literature. Moscow.1958. (translation from English)
11. Adam D. Perception, mind, memory. Mir. Moscow, 1983 (translation from English)
12. Chesset J. Introduction in psychophysiology. Moscow. Mir. 1961 (translation from English).
13. Gleser W.D. The mechanism of recognition of vision image. Science, 1966. Moscow.
14. Blechman I.I. Dynamic systems. Science, 1971.
15. Blechman I.I. Dynamic system in technique and nature. Science, 1981.
16. Walter G. The Living Brain W.W.Norton, NY, 1963

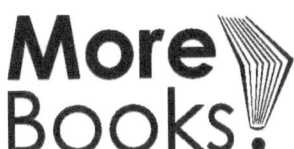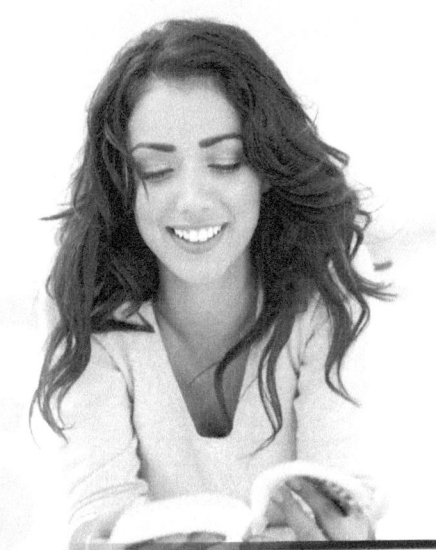

I want morebooks!

Buy your books fast and straightforward online - at one of the world's fastest growing online book stores! Environmentally sound due to Print-on-Demand technologies.

Buy your books online at
www.get-morebooks.com

Kaufen Sie Ihre Bücher schnell und unkompliziert online – auf einer der am schnellsten wachsenden Buchhandelsplattformen weltweit!
Dank Print-On-Demand umwelt- und ressourcenschonend produziert.

Bücher schneller online kaufen
www.morebooks.de

OmniScriptum Marketing DEU GmbH
Heinrich-Böcking-Str. 6-8
D - 66121 Saarbrücken
Telefax: +49 681 93 81 567-9

info@omniscriptum.com
www.omniscriptum.com

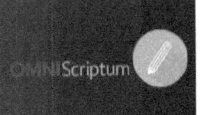

www.ingramcontent.com/pod-product-compliance
Lightning Source LLC
Chambersburg PA
CBHW031544210526
45464CB00003B/1138